NEVER AGAIN

The Untold History of Human Zoos, Scientific Racism, and the Fight for Human Dignity

By

RICHARD LOGRO PhD, RN

Clarksburg, Maryland

2026

Never Again

The Untold History of Human Zoos, Scientific Racism, and the Fight for Human Dignity

This book is a work of historical nonfiction. Every effort has been made to ensure the accuracy of the information presented through careful research and the consultation of historical sources available at the time of writing. Interpretations, analyses, and conclusions are those of the author.

Some historical language, quotations, and descriptions reproduced in this book reflect the attitudes and terminology of the periods discussed. They are included solely for historical accuracy and educational purposes and do not represent the views of the author or publisher.

The purpose of this work is to educate, preserve historical memory, and promote a deeper understanding of human dignity, ethics, and the consequences of racism, colonialism, and dehumanization.

First Edition

Printed in the United States of America

DEDICATION

To the countless men, women, and children whose names history overlooked, whose humanity was denied, and whose lives were reduced to spectacles for the amusement of others.

May this book honor your memory, restore a measure of the dignity that was taken from you, and ensure that your stories are never forgotten.

And to all who continue to defend the dignity, equality, and humanity of every person—may we never again allow curiosity, prejudice, or power to overshadow compassion and justice.

"History remembers the crowds that came to watch. This book remembers the people they came to see."

———Richard Logro PhD., RN

ACKNOWLEDGEMENTS

Unveiling uncomfortable truths through historical non-fiction demands meticulous investigation and professional endurance, alongside the unwavering encouragement and direction of numerous people and organizations. I am profoundly thankful to everyone who helped bring this book to life

First and foremost, I offer my profound thanks to my beloved wife, Mariel, whose unwavering love, emotional grounding, and constant encouragement sustained me through the long hours of archival investigation, writing, and reflection. To my daughters, thank you for your boundless joy, patience, and understanding when your father's mind was distant among the historical texts. Your presence is my greatest inspiration.

I am deeply indebted to the historians, archivists, librarians, and curators whose tireless work preserving primary sources, medical ledgers, photographs, and institutional records made the uncovering of this hidden history possible. Special appreciation is extended to the academic and professional communities in healthcare and anthropology who continue to champion bioethical standards, cultural humility, and the absolute protection of human dignity.

To my colleagues, mentors, and readers who engaged in early discussions regarding the intersection of clinical ethics and historical trauma, your insights sharpened the perspective of this work. Finally, to the memory of those whose lives and struggles fill these pages—may this book serve as an enduring testament to your resilience, ensuring that your stories are never forgotten and that your inherent dignity is forever honored.

TABLE OF CONTENTS

Author's Foreword

There are stories in history that are remembered because they celebrate human achievement, and there are stories that endure because they remind us of humanity's greatest failures. This book belongs to the latter.

For many years, I believed that the public exhibition of human beings was little more than an isolated footnote in history. The deeper I researched, however, the more I realized that it was a global phenomenon sustained by governments, scientific institutions, museums, world fairs, and millions of ordinary visitors. Men, women, and children were displayed behind fences and in constructed villages, not because they had committed crimes, but because they were considered objects of curiosity, evidence of racial theories, and symbols of imperial power.

As a registered nurse, I approached this history with a perspective shaped by healthcare ethics and the unwavering belief that every person possesses inherent dignity. While historians have carefully documented the political and colonial dimensions of human exhibitions, I found myself asking questions rooted in compassion and clinical practice. What physical suffering did these individuals endure? What emotional trauma accompanied life under constant public scrutiny? How did respected institutions justify treating human beings as exhibits rather than as people worthy of care and respect? These questions became the foundation of this work.

This book is not written to condemn the past without understanding it. Instead, it seeks to examine how prejudice, pseudoscience, economic ambition, and public acceptance combined to create one of history's most disturbing institutions. It also challenges us to consider whether the attitudes that made such exhibitions possible have truly disappeared or have merely taken different forms.

Throughout these pages, you will encounter stories of injustice, exploitation, resilience, and courage. You will meet individuals whose names deserve to be remembered not as exhibits, but as human beings with families, cultures, dreams, and identities that could never be confined by the cages built around them.

If this book accomplishes anything, I hope it encourages readers to look beyond historical events and recognize the enduring importance of empathy, cultural humility, and human dignity. History cannot be changed, but it can be remembered honestly. By remembering, we honor those who suffered, acknowledge the failures of our institutions, and strengthen our commitment to ensuring that no human being is ever again reduced to an object of curiosity or spectacle.

Thank you for taking this journey with me. May these pages deepen your understanding of the past and reinforce the timeless truth that every human life possesses equal worth and deserves unwavering respect.

Richard Logro Ph.D., RN

PREFACE

History is often remembered through the triumphs of nations, the achievements of explorers, and the progress of science. Yet beneath those celebrated narratives are stories that remained hidden for generations of individuals whose humanity was denied in the name of curiosity, commerce, and scientific inquiry. This book is dedicated to bringing one of those forgotten histories into the light.

The existence of human exhibitions, sometimes referred to as "human zoos," remains one of the least understood chapters of modern history. During the nineteenth and early twentieth centuries, thousands of Indigenous men, women, and children from Africa, Asia, the Americas, and the Pacific Islands were transported across the world and placed on public display before millions of spectators. They were exhibited in zoological parks, world fairs, colonial expositions, museums, and ethnological villages under the guise of education, anthropology, and entertainment.

As I began researching this subject, I quickly realized that this history extends far beyond the exhibition grounds themselves. It is a story of colonialism, scientific racism, institutional complicity, economic exploitation, and the gradual erosion of human dignity. More importantly, it is a story about real people whose identities, cultures, and lives deserve to be remembered with honesty and respect.

My background as a registered nurse profoundly influenced the way I approached this work. While historians often examine political movements, economic systems, and cultural change, healthcare teaches us to see the individual behind every statistic. Throughout my research, I found myself asking questions that medical professionals naturally ask: What diseases did these individuals endure after long sea voyages? How did malnutrition, unfamiliar climates, and infectious illnesses affect them? What emotional trauma resulted from living every day under the gaze of strangers? Those questions became essential to understanding not only the historical events but also their human consequences.

This book has been written from extensive historical research, including archival documents, contemporary newspapers, scholarly publications, institutional records, and firsthand accounts whenever available. Every effort has been made to present the historical evidence accurately while acknowledging that some voices were lost because those who suffered were seldom given the opportunity to record their own experiences. Where possible, this work seeks to restore those voices and recognize their humanity.

The purpose of this book is neither to sensationalize the past nor to condemn previous generations without understanding the historical context in which they lived. Instead, it seeks to examine how respected institutions, including governments, museums, universities, scientific organizations, and even the medical community—became participants in systems that treated human beings as objects rather than as people deserving dignity and respect.

Although the physical cages and exhibition grounds have disappeared, the ethical questions they raise remain deeply relevant. How do societies justify the unequal treatment of others? How can science be misused to support prejudice? What responsibilities do professionals, educators, and ordinary citizens bear when confronted with injustice? These are not merely historical questions; they continue to challenge every generation.

It is my hope that this book encourages readers to look beyond the spectacle and see the people whose lives were forever changed by these exhibitions. By remembering their stories, we honor their humanity and reaffirm a principle that should never be compromised: every person, regardless of race, culture, nationality, or circumstance, possesses inherent dignity and equal worth.

May this work serve not only as a historical account but also as a reminder that the lessons of the past are meaningful only if they shape the conscience of the present.

Richard Logro PhD., RN

Part 1

When Human Became Exhibits

Chapter 1

The Day Humanity Entered the Cage

History often remembers wars, revolutions, and the rise and fall of nations, yet some of its darkest chapters unfolded quietly, hidden beneath the applause of ordinary crowds. At the dawn of the twentieth century, the Western world celebrated an age of unprecedented discovery, industrial might, and technological marvel. Great cities competed to build magnificent museums, sprawling botanical gardens, grand zoological parks, and monumental international expositions that promised to educate the public about distant lands, exotic flora, and unfamiliar cultures.

Scientific progress was celebrated as the ultimate hallmark of civilization, while colonial empires expanded rapidly across continents under the banner of exploration, commerce, and enlightenment. Behind the elegant neoclassical architecture, polished museum exhibits, and lofty promises of public education, however, existed a deeply disturbing reality that many visitors failed—or deliberately refused—to recognize human beings had become exhibits.

To modern readers living in an era defined by international human rights frameworks, bioethical oversight, and universal standards of dignity, the idea that thousands of men, women, and children were placed on public display sounds almost impossible. Yet between the late nineteenth and early twentieth centuries, millions of visitors across Europe and the United States purchased tickets to observe Indigenous people displayed in reconstructed villages, fenced compounds, open-air theaters, and zoological settings.

They came from Africa, Asia, the Americas, the Philippines, and the Pacific Islands. They were expected to perform daily routines, demonstrate traditional crafts, and satisfy the public's insatiable fascination with what newspapers, entrepreneurs, and scientists of the era described as primitive races. What contemporary visitors considered innocent entertainment, imperial education, or harmless curiosity was the public exhibition of living human beings whose fundamental dignity, autonomy, and humanity had been stripped away for the sake of spectacle and profit.

The Architecture of Spectacle and Global Scale

This period was dominated by an intoxicating convergence of industrial capitalism, aggressive imperialism, and pseudoscientific racial theories. As European powers and the United States carved up vast portions of the globe, governments and commercial promoters sought ways to justify colonial expansion to domestic populations through the benevolent language of the civilizing mission.

World fairs and international expositions served as the premier stages for this ideological theater. Beginning with the Great Exhibition of 1851 in London's Crystal Palace and expanding through subsequent expositions in Paris, Chicago, Buffalo, Omaha, and St. Louis, these colossal events drew tens of millions of visitors. Within these meticulously constructed environments, human beings from colonized regions were relocated thousands of miles from their homes and forced to live under microscopic public scrutiny.

Cities such as Hamburg, Antwerp, London, and Paris operated as the financial and logistical epicenters of this transnational trade. In Hamburg, animal dealer Carl Hagenbeck revolutionized the industry by introducing *völkerschauen* (peoples' shows), realizing that displaying animals alongside the human beings who shared their native geographies dramatically increased profits. By the time of the 1889 Paris Exposition Universelle, which featured a massive *Village Nègre* drawing over twenty-eight million visitors, human zoos had become a massive, highly organized global industry.

The Global Logistics of Human Commodification

The procurement and transport of human beings for exhibition required the coordinated efforts of commercial booking agencies, shipping cartels, colonial administrative bureaus, and local native brokers.

- **The Supply Chain:** Specialized booking agencies in London, Antwerp, Hamburg, Marseille, and New York maintained permanent offices that monitored political instability, economic distress, and famine conditions. Interlocutors in colonized territories exploited local economic distress caused by colonial land expropriation and head taxes, offering cash advances or promises of regular employment to desperate families.
- **Transoceanic Voyage:** Transported across oceans in cramped steerage compartments, travelers were frequently listed on ship manifests alongside livestock, agricultural produce, and manufactured goods. The journey served as a brutal initial crucible of physical distress, marked by seasickness, malnutrition, and rapid climatic shock.
- **Legal Dispossession:** Upon disembarking in host ports, agents routinely confiscated passports, travel tickets, and identification papers under the pretext of safekeeping. Deprived of documentation, foreign currency, and legal recourse, stranded performers were rendered legally invisible and entirely defenseless against abuse.

Spatial Control and the Panoptic Gaze

The physical layout of ethnological villages, anthropological reservations, and zoological enclosures was directly informed by the panoptic principle—an architectural design that rendered the inmate continuously visible while denying them any reciprocal view of the observer.

In major expositions, physical boundaries were absolute. Visitors moved freely along elevated wooden boardwalks, paved concourses, and designated viewing platforms, looking down into sunken compounds where the exhibited people lived. This spatial hierarchy placed the spectator in the position of absolute authority.

- **The Eradication of Private Space:** Simulated native huts and encampments were deliberately constructed with open fronts or low fences. Families cooked over open fires, washed clothes, tended to crying infants, and slept on mats under the unblinking, unyielding gaze of thousands of strangers daily.
- **The Compulsion of Performance:** Promoters demanded a continuous simulation of "primitive" life. If an individual sat quietly reading a book, sewing, or resting out of view, guards or managers intervened to force them back into public sight.
- **Sensory Assault:** The cacophony of brass bands, steam calliopes, hawking barkers, roaring animals from nearby menageries, and tens of thousands of daily visitors created an environment of chronic sensory overload and sleep deprivation.

The Convergence of Science and Showmanship

The longevity and cultural legitimacy of human exhibitions rested upon the active, enthusiastic participation of the academic and scientific communities. During an era when Western scientific disciplines were aggressively seeking professional authority, anthropology, ethnology, and physical anthropology found an invaluable laboratory within the exhibition compounds.

University professors, museum curators, and cranial researchers viewed living human exhibits not as human beings deserving of ethical consideration, but as accessible biological specimens. Armed with standardized anthropometric instruments—craniometers to measure skull volume, sliding calipers to calculate facial angles, goniometers for joint mobility, and color charts to catalog skin pigmentation—researchers subjected exhibited individuals to exhaustive, invasive examinations.

- **Legitimization:** When a prominent professor endorsed an exhibition as a vital educational undertaking, it reassured the moral conscience of the middle-class public, transforming voyeurism into intellectual enrichment.
- **The Production of Pseudoscience:** Extracted data was published in prestigious academic journals and presented at international congresses, providing the empirical veneer that justified colonial expansion, systemic labor extraction, and racial segregation.

The Clinical Realities of the Encampment: Epidemiology and Public Health

Viewing these historical events through the lens of healthcare and clinical epidemiology reveals a stark physiological reality: the human body pushed past its biological limits by commercial enterprise.

- **Climatic and Environmental Shock:** Transporting individuals from tropical or isolated island ecosystems to damp, polluted northern industrial cities subjected their neuroendocrine systems to immense stress.
- **Epidemiological Vulnerability:** Possessing no acquired immunity to prevalent urban microbes, exhibited individuals contracted airborne pathogens like *Mycobacterium tuberculosis*, influenza viruses, and streptococcal strains with alarming speed.
- **Nutritional Deprivation:** Standard food rations were selected for low cost rather than nutritional completeness, leading to rapid weight loss, muscle wasting, and metabolic collapse.
- **Suppression of Clinical Care:** Exhibition promoters actively concealed infectious outbreaks from the public, hiding sick performers in back-alley shacks or makeshift infirmaries to prevent panic and protect ticket sales, thereby transforming treatable illnesses into fatal emergencies.

The Complicity of the Press and Popular Culture

Newspapers, illustrated magazines, and sensational adventure periodicals functioned as the primary ideological transmission belts between the exhibition compounds and the wider public, actively manufacturing the cultural consent required to sustain them.

- **The Weaponization of Headlines:** Articles utilized dehumanizing vocabulary, describing human beings as "specimens," "curiosities," "missing links," or "savages," while breathlessly hyping the theatrical illusion of wildness.
- **The Erasure of Voice:** Interviews were filtered through partisan interpreters, heavily altered, or fabricated, systematically omitting expressions of homesickness, grief, or a desire to return home.
- **The Photographic Gaze:** The advent of cheap halftone printing allowed households to flood with staged photographs of exhibited people posing with spears or in front of fake jungle backdrops, anchoring racial hierarchies deep within domestic life.

The Pathology of Indifference and the Bystander Effect

How did ordinary citizens—thousands of everyday people who considered themselves civilized, moral, and deeply religious—

walk through exhibition gates, stare at caged human beings, and feel no moral revulsion?

The answer lies in the insidious power of cultural conditioning. Decades of media saturation and pseudoscientific instruction ensured that when visitors investigated a fenced compound, they did not see a mother, a father, a son, or a daughter whose life possessed infinite value. They saw an abstraction—a living artifact of a bygone evolutionary age. This psychological distancing allowed ordinary families to treat human beings as tourist attractions, entirely blind to the moral failure unfolding before them.

Voices of Resistance and Human Agency

Despite the overwhelming institutional power arrayed behind human exhibitions, these spectacles were never accepted without challenge. A rigorous examination of the historical record reveals a continuous, courageous narrative of resistance, negotiation, and the stubborn preservation of human agency.

- **Tactical Non-Compliance:** Performers frequently weaponized passive resistance, subtly altering routines, introducing elements of satire, or performing with a deliberate lack of enthusiasm to disrupt the theatrical illusion of primitive savagery.
- **Collective Bargaining:** Recognizing their irreplaceable value as the primary attraction, several troupes organized labor strikes, refusing to leave their quarters until

management agreed to better food rations, increased pay, or rest-day excursions.

- **Legal and Consular Appeals:** Exhibited individuals sought out sympathetic journalists, foreign consuls, or local religious leaders to petition for the fulfillment of broken contracts, safe return travel, or immediate release. In 1906, when Ota Benga was displayed at the Bronx Zoo, New York's Black clergy and community leaders mobilized immediate public outrage that forced the zoo to back down.
- **Cultural Solidarity:** Communities maintained internal social bonds by speaking native languages out of earshot of guards, practicing secret traditions, sharing stories of home, and caring for one another's sickness with profound compassion.

The Unbroken Thread of Ethics and Empathy

Reflecting upon this history from the perspective of modern nursing, medicine, and bioethics, the lessons resonate far beyond the confines of historical scholarship. The transition from human exhibitions to contemporary bioethics represents a hard-won realization that human dignity is absolute, non-negotiable, and entirely independent of race, nationality, social status, or utility to others.

Modern clinical practice rests upon the foundational pillars of informed consent, patient autonomy, cultural humility, and compassionate advocacy. Every healthcare provider takes an implicit professional oath to protect the vulnerable, respect the intrinsic worth of every individual, and resist any institutional pressure that reduces a human being to a mere case number, a research specimen, or an object of administrative convenience.

The physical cages of the world's fairs and zoological parks have long since vanished into history. Yet the underlying human questions they raised remain powerfully and urgently relevant to modern society. As we examine this record, we are reminded that the erosion of human dignity never begins with overt violence; it begins with the quiet, passive acceptance of ideas, language, and cultural attitudes that divide human populations into those who deserve compassion and autonomy, and those who do not.

The Legacy of Remains: Repatriation and the Long Journey Home

When the turnstiles stopped spinning, the world's fairs closed their gates, and the temporary encampments were bulldozed into memory, a haunting material legacy was left behind in the basements and vaults of Western institutions. The tragedy of the human exhibition era did not end when the tents were struck; for many individuals who perished far from their ancestral homes, the nightmare extended into death itself.

During the height of the exhibition era, human remains—collected from performers who succumbed to tuberculosis, pneumonia, or stress-induced metabolic collapse in foreign hospitals—were frequently diverted from proper burials. Instead of being returned to grieving families, bodies were transferred to university medical departments, municipal anatomical institutes, and natural history museums. Skulls were boiled, articulated skeletons were wired together for classroom instruction, and brain tissue samples were cataloged and stored in glass jars to serve as physical trophies of pseudoscientific racial theories.

For decades, these ancestral remains rested quietly in museum drawers across Europe and the United States, treated as cataloged property rather than human beings. It is only through the relentless, generational advocacy of descendant communities, Indigenous rights organizations, and ethically conscious historians that a slow, painful process of reckoning has begun.

Repatriation movements have forced major institutions to confront their colonial archives, returning the remains of ancestors to their homelands for proper, culturally respectful burials. Yet thousands of artifacts and remains still await identification and return, serving as a silent indictment of an era when science and commerce treated human mortality as raw material.

The Architecture of Historical Amnesia

Following the mid-twentieth-century dismantling of the last human zoos—spurred by shifting global politics, post-war human rights declarations, and the moral revulsion sparked by the atrocities of World War II—Western cultural institutions engaged in a defensive process of historical amnesia.

World's fair grounds were transformed back into public parks, university laboratories scrubbed their anthropometric collections from active display, and popular memory quietly buried the reality that millions of citizens had once paid admission to stare at caged human beings. Textbooks glossed over the era as an eccentric, bygone manifestation of early anthropological curiosity, entirely omitting the coercion, the epidemiological devastation, and the profound moral failure of the institutions involved.

This collective forgetting was not accidental. Societies prefer to view their historical progression as a steady, unbroken march toward enlightenment, editing out the chapters that reveal systemic cruelty, institutional complicity, and scientific racism.

For modern healthcare professionals, researchers, and educator, breaking through this historical amnesia is a vital necessity. Understanding how ordinary municipal governments, respected universities, and celebrated scientists could seamlessly normalize the commodification of human beings shatters the comforting illusion that institutional prestige is an automatic guarantee of ethical integrity.

The Vigilance of the Healer's Lens

As we close this foundational examination of the day humanity entered the cage, the narrative returns full circle to the perspective of clinical care and professional ethics.

The transition from the human exhibition compounds of the nineteenth century to the modern bioethical frameworks of the twenty-first century was not a gift bestowed by benevolent institutions. It was forged through the exposure of past atrocities and the courageous resistance of those who refused to accept the dehumanization of their communities.

For the modern nurse and healthcare provider, this history acts as an unyielding sentinel at the gate of practice. It provides a permanent, sobering reminder of how easily the slippery slope of "othering" begins:

- **The Seduction of Utility:** Whenever human beings are evaluated primarily by their utility, whether as economic units, labor output, administrative conveniences, or research subjects—the foundational respect for human dignity is compromised.
- **The Weaponization of Authority:** When professional authority, scientific terminology, or cultural consensus are invoked to justify differential treatment, clinicians must remain vigilant against the quiet erosion of patient advocacy and human rights.
- **The Danger of Bystander Silence:** The historical reality of millions of spectators walking past fenced human beings without a word of protest reminds us that ethical failure is sustained just as much by passive indifference as it is by active malice.

The physical cages of the world's fairs and zoological parks have vanished into history. Yet the underlying human impulses that constructed them—the temptation to categorize the vulnerable, to exploit human difference for spectacle, and to look away from suffering in the name of persistent hazards in human society.

To study this history is to accept a profound professional responsibility: to ensure that human dignity remains absolute, fiercely protected, and forever beyond the reach of any system that seeks to reduce a person to an exhibit.

The Institutional Echo: Manifestations in Modern Systems

While the explicit, ticketed spectacles of nineteenth-century human zoos have been relegated to the archives of history, the underlying mechanisms of objectification, systemic paternalism, and voyeurism did not simply vanish. Instead, they evolved, migrating quietly into modern institutions, healthcare systems, administrative policies, and global development frameworks.
To trace the lineage of the human exhibition era is to recognize how easily institutional power can slip into practices that reduce human lives to data points, administrative burdens, or passive subjects of study.

- **The Data Subject vs. The Human Person:** In contemporary bureaucratic, corporate, and healthcare environments, individuals are frequently translated into alphanumeric codes, billing categories, and clinical metrics. While data collection is essential for modern operations, the administrative drift toward viewing people exclusively through the lens of utility mirrors the early anthropological reduction of human beings to measurable specimens.
- **The Paternalistic Gaze in Public Health:** Historically, colonial administrations justified human exhibitions under the benevolent guise of education and uplift. In modern global health and community interventions, parallel

paternalism can emerge when programs are designed *for* populations rather than *with* them—imposing external solutions that ignore local agency, cultural context, and self-determination.

- **The Spectacle of Vulnerability:** Contemporary media, digital platforms, and humanitarian fundraising campaigns sometimes fall into the trap of aestheticizing human suffering. By broadcasting images of poverty, crisis, or illness to elicit sympathy and donations, media structures can inadvertently echo the voyeuristic gaze of the past, strip individuals of their complex humanity and reducing them to objects of pity.

Recognizing these institutional echoes requires constant vigilance from modern professionals. It demands an intentional shift from paternalistic observation to collaborative partnership, ensuring that every individual, whether patient, student, or community member—is met with active respect for their autonomy and lived experience.

The Moral Imperative of Historical Memory

History is not merely a record of things that happened elsewhere to other people; it is a mirror reflecting the enduring vulnerabilities of human societies. The era of human zoos demonstrates with chilling clarity how quickly a civilization can normalize the unthinkable when systemic ideology overrides basic empathy.

When universities, municipal governments, scientific societies, and everyday citizens collaborated in the confinement and display of human beings, they operated not as fringe extremists, but as the mainstream pillars of their societies. They believed themselves to be modern, enlightened, and scientifically advanced. Their failure serves as our most potent warning.

For contemporary clinicians, educators, writers, and citizen, remembering this history is an act of moral resistance. It fortifies our collective immune system against the subtle creeping of prejudice, the normalization of systemic inequality, and the temptation to categorize fellow human beings as "other."

As we step away from the threshold of the nineteenth-century exhibition grounds and look toward the complex ethical landscapes of our own time, the central challenge remains unchanged: to look upon every human being not as an object to be observed, categorized, or used, but as an irreplaceable center of consciousness, dignity, and worth.

The Crucible of Global Consciousness: From Spectacle to Self-Determination

As we trace the trajectory from the fenced compounds of nineteenth-century expositions to the interconnected landscape of the modern world, we arrive at the ultimate historical counterweight to the exhibition era: the long, arduous rise of global self-determination. The human zoos of Europe and America did not exist in a vacuum; they were the theatrical frontispiece of a sprawling, violent colonial apparatus designed to convince domestic populations that subjugation was a natural, benevolent law of social evolution. Yet, within the very heart of these empires, and across the colonized territories themselves, the seeds of an intellectual and political counter-revolution were quietly taking root.

The dismantling of the human exhibition complex was never a voluntary concession handed down by enlightened administrators or paternalistic scientists. It was wrestled into existence by the relentless resistance of those who refused to be categorized as relics of a dying past. From the early twentieth century onward, anti-colonial leaders, international jurists, dissident journalists, and grassroots human rights advocates began to dismantle the pseudoscientific scaffolding of white supremacy. They exposed the systemic brutality hidden behind the manicured gardens of world's fairs and challenged the legal fictions that allowed sovereign human beings to be seized, transported, and displayed like livestock.

This historical awakening required a fundamental reordering of how global humanity understood dignity. It demanded that the West look past the distorting lens of imperialism and recognize that civilization is not measured by industrial tonnage, technological mastery, or military dominance, but by the radical, uncompromising protection of the vulnerable. The slow death of the human exhibition industry thus laid the groundwork for the post-World War II international human rights framework—a belated global consensus that codified what history had proven through blood and suffering: that human rights are universal, inalienable, and entirely non-negotiable.

The Contemporary Landscape of Dignity and Exploitation

To assume that the impulses underlying the human exhibition era have been permanently eradicated would be a dangerous historical error. While the physical cages, ticketed anthropological villages, and explicit *völkerschauen* have vanished from our public parks, the underlying psychological mechanisms—the insatiable appetite for exoticized spectacle, the utilitarian commodification of human difference, and the systemic distancing of the "other"—have simply mutated to fit the digital and globalized architecture of the twenty-first century.

In our current era, the theater of exploitation has migrated from the world's fair midway to the invisible algorithms of global digital networks, mass media, and unregulated labor markets.

- **The Digital Panopticon and Poverty Tourism:** Modern digital platforms often replicate the dynamic of the elevated boardwalk. Through sensationalized media coverage, poverty porn, and unvarnished digital voyeurism, vulnerable communities in the Global South or economically depressed regions are frequently packaged for consumption by affluent audiences. The digital "like," share, and view can function as a modern iteration of the spectator's gaze—turning distant human suffering into passive entertainment, trending content, or an object of transient charity without ever restoring structural autonomy to the individuals being viewed.

- **Globalized Labor Extraction:** The modern global supply chain often relies on invisible, highly precarious labor forces operating in distant industrial zones, agricultural fields, and informal economies. When workers are stripped of labor rights, subjected to hazardous environments, and isolated from legal protections, they are effectively treated as expendable instruments of production rather than human beings with inherent worth. The logic that viewed colonized populations as raw materials for imperial profit finds a modern echo in any economic system that prioritizes output over human life.
- **The Biomedical and Data Frontier:** As artificial intelligence, big data analytics, and global biotechnology reshape the landscape of modern medicine, new ethical fault lines emerge. The extraction of genetic data, clinical trial participation without fully realized informed consent in vulnerable populations, and the algorithmic profiling of marginalized communities remind us that the temptation to treat human lives as mere data points or biological specimens remains an active hazard.

Recognizing these modern manifestations requires a profound, unyielding cultural and professional vigilance. It challenges us to interrogate the systems we participate in daily, ensuring that efficiency, profit, and administrative convenience never supersede our fundamental duty to honor human dignity.

The Healer's Ultimate Mandate: Guardianship of the Vulnerable

For the clinician, the nurse, the educator, and the advocate, this sweeping historical exploration converges upon a single, inescapable professional mandate. Healthcare is, at its very core, an ethical enterprise. It operates in the sacred, fragile space where one human being entrusts their body, their fears, and their dignity to the care of another.

When we look back at the historical tragedy of human exhibitions, the individuals who stood behind wooden fences while thousands stared uncomprehending—we are forced to confront the ultimate failure of empathy. That failure was sustained by a profound breakdown in moral imagination. The spectators could not see the humanity of the exhibited because their culture had taught them to see only categories, races, and specimens.

As healthcare professionals and guardians of public health, our daily work is an active, living antidote to that historical failure. Every clinical interaction is an opportunity to dismantle the remnants of the objectifying gaze.

- **Active Presence:** To truly see a patient not as a diagnosis, a bed number, or a statistical metric, but as an irreplaceable center of consciousness with a unique history, family, and inner life.
- **Uncompromising Advocacy:** To stand as an ethical shield between the vulnerable and any institutional system that

seeks to reduce human value to economic utility or administrative efficiency.

- **Cultural Humility:** To approach every individual with deep respect for their lived experience, rejecting paternalism in favor of genuine, collaborative partnership in care.

The cages of the past remind us how fragile civilization is, and how quickly the boundaries of empathy can contract under the pressure of institutional ideology. Yet the history of human resistance reminds us just as powerfully that dignity cannot be permanently extinguished. It survives in the quiet acts of solidarity, the stubborn defense of human rights, and the unwavering commitment of those who refuse to look away.

As we turn the page from this foundational exploration of our shared history, we carry forward a renewed clarity of purpose. The past is not merely a record of where we have been; it is a compass pointing toward the vigilance required of us today, ensuring that no human being is ever again reduced to an exhibit.

The Threshold of Awakening: The Lasting Mandate of the Healer

As we stand at the threshold where history intersects with our present reality, the journey through the dark corridors of the human exhibition era leaves us with an indelible moral imprint.

We have traversed the grand avenues of nineteenth-century expositions, walked the perimeter of the fenced compounds in Hamburg, Paris, and St. Louis, and confronted the chilling convergence of pseudoscientific exploitation and commercialized spectacle. We have traced the institutional machinery that reduced breathing, and sent human beings to cataloged specimens, and we have witnessed the quiet, persistent resilience of those who resisted their erasure.

Yet, this historical exploration was never merely an exercise in archival documentation. It is an urgent, living meditation on the nature of human dignity and the fragility of empathy.

When the last exhibition gates closed and the wooden boardwalks were dismantled, humanity did not automatically shed the impulses that constructed them. The temptation to categorize, to commodify, and to look away from the suffering of the vulnerable remains an enduring shadow across human institutions. Whether manifest in the cold abstraction of modern data systems, the paternalistic dynamics of global development, or the subtle erosion of patient autonomy in complex healthcare bureaucracies, the ghost of the exhibition hall still haunts our systems.

For the modern healer, the educator, the writer, and the citizen, this history demands an active, daily resistance. It calls upon us to recognize that ethics is not a passive state, but an unyielding practice of radical presence. To care for another human being—whether in the busy corridors of a modern school clinic, the pages of historical research, or the quiet intimacy of bedside nursing—is to actively reject the objectifying gaze. It is a commitment to see the individual not as a case, a metric, or an exhibit, but as an infinite universe of worth, memory, and sacred potential.

The cages of the past are relics of a closed chapter, but the responsibility they impose upon us is timeless. As we conclude this foundational inquiry, we carry forward the sober realization that the defense of human dignity is never finished. It requires our constant vigilance, our deepest empathy, and our unwavering refusal to let any human being ever stand alone behind the fence again.

Chapter 2

The Empire's Stage

Colonial Expansion and the 1904 St. Louis World's Fair

When the gates of the Louisiana Purchase Exposition opened in St. Louis, Missouri, in the spring of 1904, visitors were greeted by a sprawling metropolis of neoclassical plaster palaces known as the "White City." Designed to commemorate the centennial of the 1803 land acquisition that doubled the geographic size of the United States, the fair was officially billed as a celebration of human progress, industrial ingenuity, and democratic expansion. Yet beneath the veneer of technological celebration lay a massive, federally orchestrated exercise in imperial propaganda.

The turn of the twentieth century marked a pivotal geopolitical turning point for the United States. Following the Spanish-American War of 1898, the nation had seized overseas territories in the Caribbean and the Pacific, acquiring Puerto Rico, Guam, and the Philippine archipelago, while simultaneously annexing the independent Kingdom of Hawaii. This sudden leap into overseas imperialism ignited fierce domestic debates regarding whether the U.S. should govern distant, non-white populations without their consent. Expansionists argued that these populations were unready for self-governance and required American "tutelage," while anti-imperialists condemned the acquisition as a betrayal of core democratic principles.

To resolve this ideological conflict in the court of public opinion, the organizers of the St. Louis Exposition—working in close coordination with the Department of War, the Department of the Interior, and the Smithsonian Institution—turned to anthropology as an instrument of statecraft. Under the leadership of William John McGee, a prominent ethnologist and director of the fair's Department of Anthropology, the exposition dedicated unprecedented space and financial resources to human displays. McGee did not view these exhibits as mere carnival sideshows; he conceptualized them as an empirical, living demonstration of social evolution that would visually justify American imperial policy to millions of domestic voters.

Bureaucratic Mobilization of the Philippine Reservation

The crown jewel of this anthropological enterprise was the Philippine Reservation, an unprecedented forty-seven-acre compound established on the exposition grounds. Funded by a congressional appropriation of over one million dollars and placed under the direct administrative control of the newly established Bureau of Insular Affairs, the Philippine exhibit was designed to showcase the diverse ethnic groups inhabiting the newly conquered archipelago.

To populate this massive compound, the U.S. military and civilian colonial administrators—including William Howard Taft, then-Governor-General of the Philippines—scoured the islands to recruit, coerce, or transport over one thousand Indigenous and non-Indigenous Filipinos to St. Louis. The logistical undertaking rivaled a military deployment:

Transoceanic Transport: Recruits were loaded onto U.S. Army transport ships and commercial liners, enduring weeks of grueling maritime travel across the Pacific and North American continent.

Geographic and Cultural Diversity: The reservation was meticulously compartmentalized to display a hierarchy of "civilizational advancement." It featured compounds for the Visayan and Tagalog Christianized groups, the Muslim Moros of Mindanao, the Bagobo and Negrito groups, and the Igorot communities of the northern Luzon cordilleras.

The Construction of Authenticity: Under the supervision of military engineers and ethnologists, authentic building materials—bamboo, nipa palm, and timber—were imported or replicated to construct traditional villages, complete with defensive stockades, rice paddies, and weaving sheds.

The underlying political message was broadcast with calculated clarity: the diverse peoples of the Philippines were arrayed along a spectrum from "savagery" to "incipient civilization." By placing these groups on display under the watchful eyes of American soldiers and administrators, the exposition communicated a powerful visual narrative to the American public. It argued that the inhabitants were decades, if not centuries, away from self-rule, thereby transforming colonial subjugation into a moral and humanitarian obligation.

The Igorot Experience: Sensationalism and Bodily Reduction

Among the various groups brought to St. Louis, the Igorot peoples from the rugged mountainous interior of Luzon became the primary focus of public fascination and sensationalist media coverage. Known for their distinct cultural traditions, agricultural practices, and warrior ethos, the Igorot were thrust into an environment that fundamentally distorted their identity for public consumption.

Fair promoters and sensationalist journalists quickly realized that the Igorot exhibit generated the highest ticket sales and concession revenues. To maximize this commercial return, management deliberately amplified and caricatured specific cultural traits:

The Spectacle of Dietary Customs: Sensationalized newspaper reports focused obsessively on the traditional practice of dog consumption during specific ritual feasts. Promoters capitalized on this by staging daily feeding rituals that played into Victorian tropes of cannibalism and savagery, completely stripping the practice of its sacred, communal context.

Physical Display and Dress: Although Igorot attire was historically adapted to the cool, misty climate of the mountain cordilleras, promoters pressured or required participants to wear minimal traditional clothing, maximizing visual contrast with Western visitors and exposing them to the harsh elements of the Midwestern summer.

The Staging of Rituals: Traditional dances, headhunting traditions, and metallurgical crafts were wrenched from their cultural timelines and performed repetitively on command to satisfy crowds who expected a continuous theatrical display of primitive wildness.

Despite this intense objectification, historical and archival records reveal that the Igorot participants were far from passive victims. They quickly discerned their immense economic and theatrical value to the fair organizers and utilized this leverage to negotiate for better living conditions, increased financial compensation, and greater autonomy over their daily schedules. Furthermore, they maintained fierce internal solidarity, protecting their cultural integrity behind closed doors and steadfastly refusing to allow the spectacle to fully erode their personal dignity.

The Scientific Laboratory of the Fair

While popular audiences visited the Philippine Reservation for entertainment, the academic and scientific communities viewed the exposition as a vast human laboratory. William John McGee and his team of physical anthropologists established dedicated research stations within the Department of Anthropology to conduct exhaustive anthropometric surveys on the exhibited populations.

Every day, individuals from the various troupes were subjected to invasive scientific procedures:

Craniometric Measurements: Anthropologists utilized calipers and craniometers to measure skull shapes, facial angles, and cranial volumes, seeking empirical proof of racial hierarchies.

Physiological Testing: Using dynamometers, respiratory spirometers, and acoustic devices, researchers cataloged physical strength, lung capacity, and sensory thresholds.

Photographic Archiving: Standardized anthropometric photographs—front, profile, and three-quarter views against gridded backgrounds—were captured to build a permanent visual archive of racial classification.

This data was subsequently published in monographs and presented at the International Congress of Arts and Science held concurrently at the fair. By wrapping imperial propaganda in the respectable white coat of science, the academic establishment provided the intellectual justification that allowed the American public to reconcile democratic ideals at home with brutal colonial subjugation abroad.

Shaping Public Perceptions and the Imperial Consciousness

The cultural footprint of the 1904 St. Louis World's Fair extended far beyond the closing gates of December 1904. By embedding colonial policy within a framework of popular entertainment, family recreation, and scientific education, the exposition successfully shaped American public consciousness for decades to come.

Millions of visitors returned to their hometowns across the United States carrying souvenir guidebooks, stereoscopic photographs, and deeply ingrained racial stereotypes. The exhibition reinforced the paternalistic ideology of the "White Man's Burden," convincing generations of citizens that non-white populations were inherently childlike, culturally stagnant, and incapable of governing themselves without Western intervention.

For the historian, the sociologist, and the clinician, the legacy of the St. Louis World's Fair stands as a profound historical warning. It demonstrates how seamlessly the apparatus of the modern state can utilize popular culture, media sensationalism, and co-opted scientific authority to manufacture consent for empire, turning the lived experiences of vulnerable human beings into a consumable, profitable spectacle.

The Recruitment and Mobilization of the Igorot: Mechanics of Coercion and Compliance

The presence of nearly twelve hundred Filipinos on the fairgrounds was not an accident of history, but the deliberate result of a joint initiative between the U.S. War Department, the newly established Bureau of Insular Affairs, and the civilian colonial government led by William Howard Taft.

Following the brutal Philippine-American War, American colonial officials recognized that controlling the physical territory of the archipelago was insufficient; they needed to control the narrative of empire back home. The Mountain Province of Luzon, inhabited by various ethnolinguistic groups collectively referred to by American authorities as "Igorot" (a blanket term encompassing Bontoc, Ibaloi, Kalinga, Ifugao, and other related peoples), presented a unique opportunity. Unlike the Christianized populations of the lowlands, the mountain groups had fiercely resisted both Spanish and American assimilation.

Colonial administrators devised a two-pronged strategy:

The Imperial Justification: By displaying groups portrayed as unassimilated "headhunters," the U.S. government sought to demonstrate to the American electorate that the Philippines was a fractured collection of disparate tribe's incapable of self-rule. The exhibits visually argued that American military occupation and paternalistic tutelage were moral necessities to bring order and civilization to the islands.

The Agency of Recruitment: The recruitment process itself relied heavily on a combination of coercion, economic inducement, and collaboration with local intermediaries. American military officers and civilian agents—most notably Dr. Albert Ernest Jenks, chief of the ethnographic survey in the Philippines—traveled deep into the Cordillera mountains. Jenks and his agents leveraged traditional rivalries, offered substantial monthly cash wages, promised free travel, and secured the cooperation of select local leaders who were led to believe the trip was an official diplomatic or educational mission.

Archival records reveal that the contracts signed by the Igorot participants were fundamentally deceptive. Drafted in English and Spanish—languages the recruits could not read—the agreements obscured the true nature of the daily public exhibition, framing the venture as an honorable government exchange rather than a commercial entertainment contract designed for human display.

The Architecture of the Igorot Village in St. Louis

Once the Igorot contingent arrived in St. Louis after a grueling transpacific voyage and cross-country train ride, they were assigned to a dedicated compound within the forty-seven-acre Philippine Reservation. The village was deliberately constructed to evoke an atmosphere of untouched wilderness, serving as a physical manifestation of Western evolutionary theories.

The layout and daily operations of the Igorot village were meticulously engineered to satisfy the public's appetite for the exotic:

Simulated Native Habitats: Under the supervision of fair architects, traditional pine-timber and thatched-roof huts (fayu or alang) were constructed. However, these dwellings were arranged to maximize visibility from surrounding pathways and elevated viewing platforms, stripping away any concept of domestic privacy.

The Compulsion of Ritual Performance: Fair management established a rigorous daily schedule of performances. Traditional dances, gong-playing ceremonies, and metallurgical crafting were demanded on a predictable timetable to accommodate the hundreds of thousands of visitors streaming through the gates daily.

The Sensationalization of Dietary Traditions: The most damaging and sensationalized aspect of the Igorot exhibit centered around traditional dog consumption, which was practiced during specific sacred and ceremonial feasts in the Cordillera. Sensationalist journalists and fair markers seized upon this practice, advertising the village as a "dog-eating savage camp." Visitors flocked to the compound specifically at feeding times, treating a sacred cultural ritual as a grotesque sideshow attraction.

Psychological Resilience and Agency Behind the Fences

Despite the degrading conditions, constant public surveillance, and cultural distortion, historical and archival evidence underscores that the Igorot participants were active agents who continuously negotiated their circumstances and fought to preserve their dignity.

Economic Negotiation and Leverage: The Igorot participants quickly recognized that their village was the most profitable and popular attraction within the entire Philippine Reservation. When living conditions deteriorated, when extreme Midwestern weather caused widespread illness, or when promised wages were delayed, the troupe organized collective resistance. They staged work slowdowns and refused to leave their quarters until fair administrators renegotiated financial terms and improved food rations.

Cultural Preservation in Isolation: Behind closed doors and out of sight of the crowds, the community maintained deep internal solidarity. They spoke their native languages, practiced traditional storytelling, and cared for their sickness with mutual aid, establishing an emotional fortress against the dehumanizing gaze of the fairgoers.

Post-Fair Autonomy and Legal Advocacy: Following the conclusion of the exposition in December 1904, several Igorot participants refused immediate repatriation until they secured guarantees regarding their accumulated wages and safe return transit. Some members successfully utilized legal channels and the assistance of sympathetic journalists to ensure their contracts were honored in full before embarking on the long journey back to Luzon.

The history of the Igorot at the 1904 St. Louis World's Fair stands as a profound testament to the intersection of imperial exploitation and human resilience—demonstrating how individuals retained their core identity and agency even when trapped within the most sophisticated apparatus of state-sponsored objectification.

The Cultural Encounter and the Distortion of Indigenous Identity

Before their recruitment for the exposition, the Igorot—comprising diverse ethnolinguistic groups such as the Bontoc, Ifugao, Kalinga, and Ibaloi—possessed sophisticated socio-political systems, intricate terraced agricultural engineering, and rich oral traditions. Their societies were governed by communal councils, customary laws, and a profound, spiritual relationship with their ancestral lands. Yet, when these communities were transplanted to the forty-seven-acre Philippine Reservation, exposition promoters and sensationalist media reduced this rich cultural heritage down to a single, monolithic archetype: the "primitive headhunter."

The mechanics of this cultural distortion operated on multiple levels:

The Visual Binary of Modernity versus Savagery: The fairgrounds were physically engineered to contrast the neoclassical white palaces of industrial machinery and electrical engineering with the mud, thatch, and simulated wilderness of the Igorot village. This stark spatial arrangement visually reinforced the evolutionary hierarchy promoted by the fair's anthropological department, teaching visitors to view the Igorot not as contemporaries, but as living ancestors.

The Spectacle of Metallurgy and Craft: While the Igorot possessed advanced skills in blacksmithing, woodcarving, and textile weaving, these traditional arts were framed by fair commentators as the rudimentary handiwork of "stone-age craftsmen." Rather than being celebrated as master artisans, they were exhibited as curiosities demonstrating the early phases of human industrial development.

The Erasure of Historical Context: The violent realities of the ongoing Philippine-American War—during which U.S. military forces pacified the archipelago at an immense human cost—were completely erased from the fairgrounds. In their place, the exposition substituted a paternalistic narrative of benevolent assimilation, portraying the Igorot as grateful wards of the American empire who were finally being introduced to the benefits of civilization.

The Economic and Social Realities Within the Compound

Behind the theatrical facade of the village, the daily lives of the Igorot participants were governed by strict administrative control, rigorous schedules, and the relentless physical strain of continuous performance. While fair promoters reaped substantial financial rewards from gate receipts and souvenir sales, the participants experienced a reality defined by isolation and institutional surveillance.

The dietary controversy surrounding dog consumption serves as a striking example of how cultural practices were exploited for commercial gain. Within traditional Cordillera society, the consumption of dog meat was restricted to specific, highly sacred ritual occasions—such as major religious feasts, peace pacts, or healing ceremonies—carrying deep spiritual significance. Fair promoters, recognizing the sensationalist value of this practice to Victorian sensibilities, aggressively advertised the village around it. They scheduled feeding times to coincide with peak visitor hours, turning a sacred communal ritual into a daily sideshow that attracted gawking crowds and generated widespread public revulsion and moral posturing among middle-class American visitors.

Despite these indignities, the Igorot participants demonstrated remarkable resilience and internal cohesion. Archival records indicate that the community established informal governance structures within the compound to mediate internal disputes, regulate daily labor expectations, and protect vulnerable members from abusive managers. When working conditions became intolerable, such as during the brutal Midwestern heat waves that caused widespread respiratory illness, the troupe utilized collective bargaining, threatening work stoppages until exposition authorities agreed to improve food quality, provide adequate medical care, and adjust daily performance hours.

The Legacy of the Igorot Exhibit in Modern Historiography

The presence of the Igorot at the 1904 St. Louis World's Fair left a complex, painful legacy that continues to resonate in contemporary Philippine-American history and Indigenous rights advocacy. For decades, the historical memory of the exhibit was dominated by photographs, anthropological monographs, and journalistic accounts produced by the very institutions that exploited them.

In recent years, however, historians, educators, and the descendants of those who traveled to St. Louis have engaged in a vital process of historical reclamation. By examining oral histories, family archives, and official government correspondence, modern scholarship has successfully shifted the narrative. The Igorot participants are no longer viewed as passive victims of imperial curiosity, but as resilient historical actors who navigated an extraordinary transnational ordeal with remarkable dignity, preserving their cultural identity against overwhelming structural odds.

The Long Tail of Spectacle: Post-Fair Tours and the Commercialization of Identity

When the gates of the 1904 Louisiana Purchase Exposition finally closed in December 1904, the physical pavilions of the "White City" were systematically dismantled, but the machinery of human exhibition did not stop. For the Igorot and other Indigenous groups from the Philippine Reservation, the conclusion of the St. Louis World's Fair marked not a return home, but the beginning of a grueling, migratory cycle of commercial exploitation across the United States and Europe.

Enterprising managers, former military officers, and exposition officials—such as Truman Hunt and officials from the Philippine Exposition Board—recognized the immense commercial potential of the troupes. Having witnessed how effectively sensationalized presentations of culture could generate box-office revenue, these promoters formed private syndicates. They approached members of the Igorot contingent with promises of continued wages, travel, and adventure, securing contracts for nationwide touring circuits.

These post-fair tours carried the human zoo model directly into urban centers, amusement parks, and regional state fairs:

The Coney Island and Vaudeville Circuit: Troupes were integrated into commercial entertainment hubs like New York's Coney Island, urban vaudeville theaters, and exposition parks across Detroit, Chicago, and beyond. In these venues, the thin veneer of "anthropological education" was entirely stripped away, laying bare the raw, unadulterated mechanics of commercial voyeurism.

The Institutionalization of Stereotypes: Promoters relentlessly recycled the sensationalized tropes birthed in St. Louis. Advertisements and press releases continued to spotlight simulated headhunting displays and daily dog-consumption routines, cementing deep-seated, racialized caricatures of Filipinos in the American popular imagination that persisted for generations.

The Erosion of Legal Protection: Far from home, stripped of documentation, and navigating unfamiliar legal systems, touring performers often found themselves trapped by broken promises, withheld wages, and severe physical exhaustion as promoters cut costs to maximize profits.

Yet, even within these predatory commercial circuits, the performers continued to exercise at the agency where they could.

Some individuals successfully utilized local legal systems, sought the aid of sympathetic journalists or anti-imperialist leagues, or leveraged their indispensable status as performers to demand better financial terms before breaking contracts and finding their own paths back to the Philippine cordilleras.

Shaping the Imperial Imagination: The Societal Echoes

The legacy reveals how deeply public spectacles can alter the trajectory of national consciousness. By framing overseas imperial conquest through the lens of family entertainment, scientific validation, and popular amusement, the 1904 St. Louis World's Fair and its subsequent touring iterations successfully manufactured public consent for American hegemony in the Pacific.

Millions of citizens who visited the Philippine Reservation absorbed a clear, powerful ideological lesson: that governance of distant lands was not an act of territorial aggression, but a paternalistic duty owed by a superior civilization to those deemed incapable of self-rule. This cultural conditioning cast a long shadow over twentieth-century foreign policy, normalizing systems of racial hierarchy and administrative control whose consequences reverberate to this day.

The Broadening Scope of the Philippine Reservation: Beyond the Igorot

While the Igorot groups captured the primary focus of sensationalist media and popular curiosity at the 1904 St. Louis World's Fair, the forty-seven-acre Philippine Reservation was designed as a comprehensive microcosm of the entire archipelago.

To fulfill the scientific and political mandates of the exposition, federal organizers and ethnologists engineered distinct, compartmentalized compounds for several other major ethnolinguistic groups, each serving a specific rhetorical function in the overarching narrative of American imperial expansion.

The Visayan and Tagalog Villages: Positioned near the entrance of the reservation, these compounds showcased Christianized lowlanders. Exhibiting advanced masonry, European-style dress, agricultural trades, and Western musical performances, these troupes were presented as the "most civilized" elements of the archipelago. Promoters used them to demonstrate the success of prior Spanish religious and cultural conversion, while simultaneously arguing that they represented an intermediate tier requiring American political stewardship to achieve full democratic maturity.

The Moro Encampment: Representing the Muslim populations of the southern Philippines (primarily Mindanao and the Sulu Archipelago), the Moro compound was constructed to evoke an atmosphere of martial exoticism. Featuring elaborate weaponry, traditional brassware craftsmanship, and distinctive architecture, the Moro were framed by fair organizers as fierce, independent warriors who had resisted both Spanish rule and initial American incursions. Their inclusion served to justify an ongoing, heavy military presence in the southern islands under the guise of maintaining regional pacification.

The Negrito Encampment: Placed at the margins of the reservation, the small group of Negritos—indigenous forest-dwellers characterized by small stature and distinct physical features—was utilized by physical anthropologists as the ultimate anchor for the lower end of the unilinear evolutionary scale. Anthropologists subjected them to rigorous, daily anthropometric measurements, framing them as living relics of an ancient human past.

This carefully orchestrated architecture of human classification allowed the exposition to present a unified, persuasive ideological argument: the Philippines was not a cohesive nation ready for immediate independence, but a fractured mosaic of disparate peoples at varying stages of development, all urgently requiring the benevolent, stabilizing hand of American empire.

The Domestic and International Repercussions: Anti-Imperialist Pushback and Global Media

The massive scale and intense public visibility of the Philippine Reservation did not go unchallenged. Even as millions of Americans walked the fairgrounds and purchased souvenir guidebooks, a fierce ideological battle was unfolding in the national press, political circles, and anti-imperialist organizations across the United States.

Prominent anti-imperialist figures, journalists, and reform-minded intellectuals—including members of the American Anti-Imperialist League—vocalized sharp condemnations of the human exhibits. They argued that displaying foreign human beings as zoological specimens was a profound moral regression that fundamentally contradicted America's foundational democratic ideals.

The Critique of Hypocrisy: Critics highlighted the glaring contradiction between official government rhetoric—which claimed the U.S. was bringing liberty, education, and self-governance to the Philippines—and the reality of confining Filipinos behind fences to be gawked at by paying crowds.

Protests from the Islands: News of the sensationalized treatment of the Igorot and other groups eventually filtered back to the Philippines, sparking indignation among local elites, nationalist newspapers, and political leaders who viewed the exhibitions as a national humiliation designed to justify colonial subjugation.

Despite these sharp criticisms, the popular momentum of the fair overwhelmed domestic dissent. The sheer entertainment value, combined with the reassuring stamp of scientific authority provided by the Department of Anthropology, ensured that the public perception of the exhibits remained overwhelmingly celebratory. The exposition succeeded in embedding an enduring, paternalistic view of overseas populations into the American cultural consciousness, demonstrating the powerful role that institutionalized spectacle could play in shaping modern imperial policy.

The Ideological Machinery of the Empire's Stage

The St. Louis World's Fair was not merely a passive mirror of turn-of-the-century racial attitudes; it was an active, highly funded industrial laboratory where public consent for American overseas imperialism was methodically manufactured, packaged, and distributed to millions of citizens.

When the McKinley and Roosevelt administrations made the fateful decision to retain the Philippine archipelago following the conclusion of the Spanish-American War in 1898 and the brutal suppression of the subsequent Philippine-American War, they faced a profound domestic crisis of legitimacy. A republic founded on the anti-colonial principles of 1776 was suddenly transformed into an overseas colonizer ruling over millions of non-white subjects without their consent. The anti-imperialist movement—led by prominent intellectuals, industrialists, and politicians—warned that militarized expansionism would corrupt American democracy from within.

It was against this volatile political backdrop that exposition organizers, military planners, and anthropological bureaucrats formed a powerful coalition. They recognized that abstract political debates in congressional halls could be decisively short-circuited by a sensory appeal on a massive national stage. By physically bringing over one thousand Filipinos to St. Louis and placing them within a meticulously engineered landscape of evolutionary hierarchy, the federal government bypassed intellectual debate and anchored imperial ideology directly into popular entertainment, family recreation, and visual culture.

The Bureaucratic Anatomy of the Philippine Reservation: Logistics, Funding, and Military Command

The realization of the forty-seven-acre Philippine Reservation required an administrative and logistical effort that rivaled major military campaigns. The enterprise was backed by a massive congressional appropriation of one million dollars—an extraordinary sum for the era—and was placed under the direct operational command of the Bureau of Insular Affairs and the U.S. War Department.

The logistical pipeline required to source, transport, and house over one thousand individuals from diverse linguistic and geographical backgrounds across the Pacific Ocean and the North American continent demonstrated the terrifying efficiency of the modern colonial state:

The Role of Colonial Officials: High-ranking civilian and military officials in the Philippines—most notably William Howard Taft, then-Governor-General of the archipelago, and civil servants within the newly formed ethnographic survey—personally oversaw the selection and recruitment of troupes. They utilized local police networks, district governors, and tribal intermediaries to secure participants, frequently exploiting local rivalries, economic disruptions, and political vulnerabilities caused by recent warfare.

The Maritime and Overland Transit: Recruits were boarded onto military transport and commercial liners, enduring weeks of harsh maritime conditions before arriving at West Coast ports. From there, they were loaded onto specialized cross-country trains, arriving in St. Louis isolated, disoriented, and entirely dependent on the military personnel assigned to guard them.

The Compartmentalization of Identity: Once inside the reservation, the inhabitants were segregated into distinct compounds designed to mirror an evolutionary ladder. The spatial arrangement was a physical manifestation of unilinear cultural evolution: Christianized lowlanders (Visayans and Tagalogs) were housed near the entrance to represent "incipient civilization"; Muslim Moros occupied a fortified compound representing martial resistance; and the Igorot and Negrito groups were placed deeper within the grounds to symbolize the raw, uncultivated starting points of human development.

This spatial segregation was deliberately engineered to teach visitors a simple, reductive lesson: that the diverse populations of the Philippines were incapable of uniting into a modern nation-state, and that American tutelage was an absolute, humanitarian prerequisite for their eventual development.

The Micro-Politics of Daily Life Inside the Reservation

Within the confines of the Philippine Reservation, the daily lives of the participants were subjected to relentless administrative surveillance, rigid timetables, and the unyielding gaze of the paying public. The compounds were surrounded by fences, ropes, and security checkpoints, effectively turning domestic life into a permanent public performance.

For the participants, the psychological and physical toll of this existence was profound:

The Destruction of Domestic Privacy: Activities that belong to the private, restorative sphere—such as preparing family meals, nursing infants, grieving, and sleeping—were dragged into the open glare of public consumption. Visitors crowded viewing platforms, tossing food, shouting questions, and treating human beings as zoological specimens.

The Commercialization of Cultural Sacredness: The exploitation of the Igorot dog-consumption ritual stands as a prime example of how complex religious and social customs were stripped of their meaning and weaponized for box-office appeal. Promoters sensationalized the practice in daily newspapers, scheduling public feedings to maximize turnstile receipts and stoking Victorian prejudices regarding savagery and civilization.

The Environment of Exposure: The Midwestern summer climate—notoriously humid, stifling, and prone to severe storms—proved physically punishing for individuals unaccustomed to such weather. Combined with substandard rations and continuous exhaustion from mandatory performance schedules, camp inhabitants suffered from high rates of respiratory illness, gastrointestinal distress, and profound psychological burnout.

Despite these harrowing conditions, archival records consistently highlight the remarkable resilience and agency of the participants. They formed internal support networks, utilized traditional languages to create private communicative spaces inaccessible to guards, and engaged in collective labor negotiations—including work slowdowns and protests—when living conditions or pay became intolerable. They refused to let the institutional machine completely erase their humanity.

The Scientific Co-Option: Anthropometry as Imperial Justification

The ideological legitimacy of the Philippine Reservation was heavily reinforced by the fair's Department of Anthropology, directed by William John McGee. Working in tandem with physical anthropologists, ethnologists, and medical researchers, McGee transformed the human exhibits into an active scientific laboratory.

Every day, individuals from the various troupes were led to testing stations where they were subjected to invasive, pseudoscientific examinations:

Craniometric and Bodily Measurement: Researchers measured cranial vaults, facial angles, limb lengths, and skin pigmentation using calipers, goniometers, and color charts, seeking empirical validation for racial hierarchies.

Physiological Testing: Using spirometers and dynamometers, scientists cataloged physical strength, lung capacity, and sensory thresholds, publishing their findings in prestigious academic journals and presenting them at the concurrent International Congress of Arts and Science.

The Archival Fixation: Standardized anthropometric photographs were captured to build a permanent visual archive, lending the unassailable prestige of academic science to political policies designed to justify colonial subjugation, disenfranchisement, and racial segregation.

Domestic and International Repercussions: Public Perception and Anti-Imperialist Resistance

The cultural footprint of the 1904 St. Louis World's Fair extended far beyond its closing months, successfully embedding paternalistic stereotypes of overseas populations into the American consciousness for generations. Millions of visitors returned home carrying souvenir guidebooks, stereoscopic photographs, and deeply ingrained racial biases that normalized American hegemony in the Pacific.

However, this massive exercise in propaganda did not go uncontested. Anti-imperialist organizations, reform-minded journalists, and nationalist newspapers in the Philippines mounted fierce critiques, condemning the exhibitions as a moral regression that betrayed American democratic principles and humiliated the Filipino people on the global stage. Yet, the combined force of government backing, scientific endorsement, and popular entertainment proved overwhelming, cementing an imperial narrative that would shape foreign policy for decades.

The Structural Mechanics of Empire: Anthropology Days and Institutional Legacy

Organized in August 1904 by William John McGee and James E. Sullivan, head of the Department of Physical Culture, this two-day sports competition brought members of the human exhibits—including Igorot, Negrito, and other Indigenous groups from the Philippine Reservation, alongside Native Americans and African displays—into the Olympic stadium to compete in standard Western athletic events such as running, jumping, and tug-of-war.

The underlying intent of Anthropology Days was not recreational or celebratory; it was an aggressive attempt to generate empirical proof of unilinear racial evolution. Fair organizers and physical anthropologists hypothesized that non-Western peoples would universally underperform compared to white athletes, thereby scientifically validating the notion of white biological and cultural supremacy.

The Distortion of Athletic Competence: Competing without prior training, equipment, or familiarity with standardized rules, the participants were set up for systemic failure. When individuals struggled with unfamiliar sports like the shot put or pole vault, researchers recorded these moments as definitive proof of intellectual and physical inferiority.

The Manipulation of Data: Paradoxically, when individual competitors occasionally excelled—such as outperforming expectations in endurance running or agility tests dismissed these results as anomalies or attributed them to animalistic instinct rather than athletic skill.

The Final Verdict of the Arena: The event concluded with the public proclamation that "primitive" peoples possessed lower physical coordination and mental stamina, providing the mainstream American press with ready-made headlines to justify imperial paternalism, domestic segregation, and colonial subjugation.

The Human Toll: Mortality, Illness, and Structural Neglect

Behind the festive exterior of the White City and the constant stream of curious visitors, the physical toll on the inhabitants of the Philippine Reservation was devastating. Archival health records and municipal death registers document the severe human cost of uprooting over one thousand individuals and housing them in an experimental camp environment exposed to extreme environmental stressors.

Throughout the seven months of the exposition, approximately seventeen individuals—primarily from the Igorot,

Negrito, and Bontoc contingents—lost their lives within the reservation. The primary causes of mortality included:

Epidemic Vulnerability: Lacking acquired immunity to endemic midwestern pathogens, participants suffered high rates of acute respiratory infections, measles, and tuberculosis. The transition from tropical climates to the humid, volatile weather of St. Louis triggered severe pulmonary illnesses.

Nutritional and Environmental Stress: Substandard institutional rations, combined with the psychological weight of constant confinement and performance pressure, severely compromised the immune systems of the camp residents.

Institutional Cover-Ups: Exposition administrators and camp managers frequently attempted to conceal deaths and severe illnesses from the public eye, transferring dying individuals to distant city hospitals at the last moment to avoid negative publicity that might dampen ticket sales.

The Enduring Legacy

The events of the 1904 St. Louis World's Fair left a profound, multi-layered legacy that continues to influence contemporary historical understanding. By merging industrial technology, popular entertainment, federal propaganda, and pseudoscientific anthropology into a single, cohesive spectacle, the exposition demonstrated how easily a democratic society could be mobilized to support overseas empires.

The images, motion pictures, and journalistic accounts generated during the fair etched enduring, racialized caricatures into the global consciousness. Yet, looking back through the lens of modern historical analysis, the true narrative of the Philippine Reservation is not merely one of victimization. It stands as a powerful testament to the resilience, agency, and quiet defiance of individuals who navigated an unprecedented imperial ordeal, preserving their humanity and cultural dignity long after the plaster palaces of the White City crumbled into dust.

The conclusion of the St. Louis exposition did not dismantle the ideological framework of the Philippine Reservation; rather, it catalyzed its commercial replication on a national scale. Promoters and syndicate managers quickly realized that the public appetite for racialized spectacle remained voracious, prompting them to funnel former participants into a grueling network of regional state fairs, vaudeville houses, and amusement parks. In these secondary venues, the thin, academic pretense of "ethnographic education" was entirely discarded, exposing the raw, transactional nature of human exhibition. Stripped of their institutional surroundings, performers found themselves navigating an unyielding circuit of commercial voyeurism where their daily routines were commodified for profit, further entrenching harmful imperial stereotypes into the American cultural landscape long after the fairgrounds had gone dark.

As these traveling troupes traversed the urban centers and rural exhibition circuits of the United States, they inadvertently created localized friction points that challenged the tidy, paternalistic narratives constructed in St. Louis. Local newspapers in smaller towns frequently sensationalized the arrival of the performers with lurid headlines, yet these encounters also forced ordinary citizens to confront the living human cost of overseas expansion up close. In some instances, local labor unions and progressive reform groups questioned the ethics of parading foreign workers through commercial sideshows, occasionally offering informal legal aid or sanctuary to individuals attempting to break away from abusive managers. These grassroots interventions, though sporadic and frequently suppressed by local authorities, highlighted the growing domestic discomfort surrounding the industrialization of human display and foreshadowed the rising tide of anti-colonial critique that would gradually dismantle the structural viability of human exhibitions in the decades to follow.

The Institutionalization of Imperial Ideology: The Broader Administrative and Sociological Matrix

The forty-seven-acre Philippine Reservation was not merely a passive display of cultural artifacts; it was a highly organized institutional apparatus designed to resolve a fundamental contradiction at the heart of American democracy at the dawn of the twentieth century.

When the United States annexed the Philippine archipelago following the Treaty of Paris in 1898 and subsequently suppressed the armed resistance of the Philippine-American War, the nation inherited an overseas empire containing millions of non-white subjects. This sudden transition from a continental republic to an overseas colonial power provoked intense domestic opposition. Anti-imperialists argued that holding colonies violated the core tenets of the Declaration of Independence and threatened to corrupt domestic republican institutions through militarism and racial subjugation.

In response, the architects of American foreign policy—led by figures like William Howard Taft, Secretary of War Elihu Root, and ethnologists within the Smithsonian Institution—mobilized the apparatus of the federal government to construct a counter-narrative. They asserted that the inhabitants of the newly acquired territories were not yet ready for self-governance, framing colonial domination not as an act of territorial aggression, but as a benevolent, civilizing trusteeship. To make this abstract political theory palpable to the American voter, the federal government appropriated over one million dollars—an unprecedented sum for an exposition exhibit—to transport more than one thousand Filipinos across the Pacific Ocean and place them on display in St. Louis.

The Logistical Nexus and the Bureaucratic Procurement of Human Cargo

The realization of the Philippine Reservation required a vast, transnational logistical pipeline managed jointly by the U.S. Army, the Bureau of Insular Affairs, and specialized civilian agents. The recruitment process relied heavily on colonial administrators who scoured the archipelago, leveraging local political vulnerabilities, economic disruptions caused by years of warfare, and traditional tribal divisions to secure participants.

Recruitment Networks: Ethnologists such as Dr. Albert Ernest Jenks traveled deep into the Luzon cordilleras and the southern islands, negotiating with local leaders and presenting the journey under varying pretenses. While some recruits were offered attractive monthly wages or led to believe they were embarking on an official governmental delegation, others experienced varying degrees of subtle coercion and deception regarding the true nature of the daily public exhibitions.

Transoceanic Transit: Once recruited, participants were marshaled onto military transport and commercial liners, enduring weeks of grueling maritime conditions. Upon arrival at West Coast ports, they were transferred to sealed railway cars and transported across the American continent, arriving in St. Louis isolated, disoriented, and surrounded by military guards and exposition handlers.

The Spatial Hierarchy of the Compounds: Inside the reservation, the layout of the over 130 buildings were meticulously designed to mirror unilinear social evolution. Christianized lowlanders from the Visayas and Tagalog regions were placed near the entrance to represent the highest tier of "incipient civilization" achievable under prior Spanish tutelage. Moving deeper into the reservation, visitors encountered the Muslim Moro compound, which was curated to highlight martial independence and justify ongoing military pacification in Mindanao. Furthest inward lay the compounds of the Igorot and Negrito groups, positioned deliberately to represent the primordial starting points of human development.

The Reduction of Culture: The Igorot Experience Under the Microscope

Within this engineered evolutionary landscape, the Igorot groups from the northern mountains of Luzon became the primary focal point of public curiosity, sensationalist media coverage, and commercial exploitation. Their rich cultural heritage—comprising complex terraced agricultural systems, democratic village councils, and intricate customary laws—was systematically flattened into a single, marketable archetype: the "primitive headhunter."

Exposition promoters quickly recognized that sensationalism drove ticket sales. Daily routines were transformed into theatrical performances tailored to Victorian sensibilities:

The Weaponization of Dietary Customs: The traditional consumption of dog meat during sacred Cordillera rituals was seized upon by sensationalist journalists and fair barkers. By scheduling public feedings to coincide with peak visitor hours, promoters turned a solemn religious and communal rite into a grotesque daily spectacle, generating widespread public voyeurism and reinforcing racist tropes of savagery.

The Physical Toll of Exposure: The Midwestern summer climate—marked by extreme humidity, volatile storms, and fluctuating temperatures—proved physically devastating for participants accustomed to the cool, stable air of the mountain cordilleras. Combined with high-stress performance schedules and inadequate institutional support, residents suffered from high rates of acute respiratory illness, gastrointestinal distress, and profound psychological exhaustion.

The Architecture of Surveillance: Fences, ropes, and constant security patrols stripped participants of all domestic privacy. Private moments of rest, grief, and family life were exposed to the unblinking gaze of hundreds of thousands of paying spectators, turning human existence into a permanent commodity.

Agency, Resistance, and Negotiation Within the Fences

Despite the overwhelming institutional power of the exposition management and the degrading nature of the daily displays, historical and archival evidence consistently demonstrates that the Filipino participants were far from passive victims. They recognized their indispensable economic value to the fair—the Philippine Reservation was one of the most profitable attractions on the grounds—and utilized this leverage to contest their conditions.

Collective Bargaining and Work Stoppages: When living conditions deteriorated, when extreme weather caused widespread illness, or when promised wages were delayed or withheld, the troupes organized collective pushbacks. They staged work slowdowns, refused to leave their quarters, and demanded direct renegotiations with fair administrators regarding food quality, medical care, and performance hours.

The Preservation of Cultural Autonomy: Behind closed doors and out of sight of the crowds, participants maintained strict internal solidarity. They spoke their native languages, practiced traditional storytelling, and established mutual aid networks that formed an emotional fortress against the dehumanizing gaze of the fairgoers.

Post-Fair Legal Advocacy: Following the conclusion of the exposition in December 1904, many participants refused immediate repatriation until they secured guarantees regarding their accumulated wages and safe return transit. Some individuals successfully utilized local legal systems or sought the aid of sympathetic journalists to ensure their contracts were honored in full before embarking on the long journey back to the Philippines.

The Scientific Co-Option: Anthropometry and "Anthropology Days"

The ideological legitimacy of the Philippine Reservation was heavily reinforced by the fair's Department of Anthropology, directed by William John McGee. Working in tandem with physical anthropologists and medical researchers, McGee transformed the human exhibits into an active scientific laboratory where pseudoscientific methods were deployed to validate racial hierarchies.

Anthropometric Examinations: Daily, individuals from the various tropes were subjected to invasive physical measurements. Researchers utilized calipers, craniometers, and color charts to measure cranial vaults, facial angles, and limb lengths, seeking empirical proof of inherent racial differences in intelligence and capability.

Anthropology Days: In August 1904, organizers hosted a specialized two-day sports competition known as "Anthropology Days," bringing Indigenous participants into the Olympic stadium to compete in standard Western athletic events. Competing without prior training, equipment, or familiarity with standardized rules, the participants were set up for systemic failure. When individuals struggled with unfamiliar sports, researchers recorded these moments as definitive proof of intellectual and physical inferiority, publishing their findings in academic journals to justify imperial paternalism.

The Domestic Impact and the Long Shadow of Imperial Spectacle

The cultural footprint of the 1904 St. Louis World's Fair extended far beyond its closing months, successfully embedding paternalistic stereotypes of overseas populations into the American consciousness for generations. Millions of visitors returned home carrying souvenir guidebooks, stereoscopic photographs, and deeply ingrained racial biases that normalized American hegemony in the Pacific.

Furthermore, when the exposition closed, the machinery of human exhibition did not dismantle; it merely decentralized. Promoters and syndicate managers funneled former participants into a grueling network of regional state fairs, vaudeville houses, and amusement parks across North America and Europe. In these secondary venues, the thin academic pretense of "ethnographic education" was entirely discarded, exposing the raw, transactional nature of human exhibition and ensuring that the harmful caricatures forged in St. Louis persisted for decades, shaping public perception and immigration policies long after the plaster palaces of the White City had crumbled into dust.

The Sociopolitical Aftershocks in the Philippines and the Birth of Critical Historiography

While the domestic American press celebrated the Louisiana Purchase Exposition as a triumphant showcase of modern progress and benevolent paternalism, the geopolitical shockwaves registered sharply across the Pacific in the Philippine Islands. The physical exhibition of over one thousand Filipinos behind exhibition fences was perceived by the burgeoning nationalist press, local intellectuals, and political leaders in Manila not as an educational exchange, but as a deliberate and humiliating assault on national dignity. Newspapers such as El Renacimiento published scathing editorials condemning the exposition as an imperial strategy designed to convince the Western world that Filipinos were perpetual children incapable of self-governance. These critiques underscored a profound diplomatic tension: even as colonial governor-wide administrators like William Howard Taft defended the exhibits as scientific and educational necessities, the lived reality for the colonized population was one of public commodification and structural degradation.

This widening chasm between official imperial rhetoric and grassroots outrage laid the groundwork for decades of anti-colonial resistance. The indignities suffered by the Igorot, Moro, Visayan, and Negrito troupes in St. Louis became a rallying point for Filipino nationalists who argued that American occupation was fundamentally incompatible with democratic self-determination. The archival record left behind by these events—comprising official government reports, anthropological monographs, municipal police ledgers, and oral histories—has served as a vital foundation for modern historical revisionism. Today, historians, Indigenous rights advocates, and descendants of the original participants are engaged in a rigorous process of historical reclamation. They have successfully shifted the academic narrative, transforming the subjects of the 1904 exposition from passive victims of imperial voyeurism into resilient historical actors who navigated an extraordinary transnational ordeal with remarkable courage, preserving their cultural identity long after the physical structures of the White City had vanished.

The Legacy of Archival Reclamation and the Ethics of Human Display

The enduring historical weight of the 1904 St. Louis World's Fair forces a critical re-examination of how modern institutions curate, interpret, and display the cultural heritage of Indigenous and colonized peoples. For decades, the primary historical footprint of the Philippine Reservation consisted almost entirely of the administrative documents, sensationalist press clippings, and anthropometric archives produced by the very state apparatus that exploited them. This structural imbalance meant that the voices, motivations, and internal agency of the participants were systematically erased from the official historical record, leaving behind a distorted narrative that favored the perspective of the colonizer over the colonized.

In contemporary historiography, the task of archival reclamation has become a moral and academic imperative. Historians, museum curators, and the direct descendants of the Igorot, Negrito, Moro, and lowlander troupes are actively working to correct this historical distortion. By combing through oral histories, family photographs, international correspondence, and overlooked municipal records, modern research is reconstituting the individual identities behind the anthropological catalog numbers. This work transforms anonymous "specubjects" back into named historical actors with distinct families, personal aspirations, and profound resilience.

Furthermore, history serves as a foundational case study in museum ethics and anthropological practice today. It stands as a permanent institutional warning against the dangers of cultural objectification, scientific racism, and the weaponization of public exhibition for political ends. As cultural institutions worldwide continue to audit their collections, restitute ancestral remains, and decolonize their display methodologies, the ghosts of the White City remind us of the heavy ethical cost incurred whenever human lives are reduced to a consumable spectacle for the entertainment of empire.

The Persistent Echoes of 1904: Memory, Repatriation, and Modern Reckoning

The shadow cast by the Philippine Reservation extends far beyond academic monographs and museum ethics guidelines; it resonates deeply within the modern cultural consciousness of the Cordillera region and the broader Philippine diaspora. For generations, the physical artifacts, photographs, and human remains collected during the 1904 exposition remained scattered across Western institutional archives, university vaults, and private collections. These items served as silent testaments to an era when human dignity was bartered for imperial entertainment.

In recent years, descendants of the Igorot participants and indigenous rights organizations have mobilized around initiatives aimed at archival repatriation and historical truth-telling. These efforts seek to bring home the fragmented histories left behind in St. Louis—ranging from digital copies of official government documents to the return of cultural objects that were appropriated or traded away during the fair. By reclaiming these narratives, contemporary Indigenous communities are rewriting the historical record on their own terms, ensuring that the resilience and agency of their ancestors outshine the transient spectacle of the White City.

When the 1904 St. Louis World's Fair closed its gates, the paths of the Igorot participants diverged in complex and often arduous ways. While some members of the troupe were eventually repatriated back to the Luzon Cordilleras—carrying with them earned wages, manufactured goods, and altered worldviews that occasionally emphasized the value of Western education for their children—many others faced a different fate. Private syndicates and former exposition managers, recognizing the immense profit margins of human exhibitions, quickly formed commercial touring companies. These entrepreneurs locked groups of Igorot performers into extended contracts, funneling them into a grueling, decade-long migratory circuit of vaudeville theaters, amusement parks, and regional state fairs across the United States, Canada, and Europe.

Caught within these secondary touring networks, performers like Antero Cabrera navigated a transnational limbo, spending years moving back and forth between Western entertainment venues and their ancestral homes. While some individuals managed to assert their independence, seek legal recourse, or integrate into local communities abroad with the aid of sympathetic reformers, others suffered from profound physical exhaustion, cultural alienation, and psychological distress. Ultimately, the conclusion of the St. Louis exposition did not mark a clean endpoint for the Igorot participants but rather initiated a prolonged chapter of commercial displacement and survival that permanently altered personal lineages and left deep scars across the collective memory of the Cordillera peoples.

The Return and the Long Road Home: Reintegrating into the Cordillera

For those Igorot participants who finally made the long, arduous journey back to the northern mountains of Luzon, the return was rarely a simple restoration of the life they had left behind in 1904. Stepping off the coastal steamers and hiking back up the steep, mist-shrouded trails of the Cordillera, they returned to communities that had undergone significant changes under American colonial administration.

The reintegration process was marked by complex paradoxes:

Cultural Translation and Dislocation: Many returnees brought back foreign goods, manufactured tools, and a firsthand understanding of Western industrial society. However, they also carried the psychological weight of having been commodified, studied, and sensationalized as "savages" for millions of foreign spectators. Discussing the intimate realities of the exposition often proved difficult, leading many to maintain a guarded silence about their experiences across the Pacific.

Shifting Social Dynamics: Some individuals who had served as leaders or interpreters within the tropes utilized their earnings or newly forged bureaucratic connections to navigate the evolving colonial administration. Yet, this often-created internal community tensions, as traditional village hierarchies rubbed against individuals who had been co-opted, even temporarily, by the machinery of empire.

The Permanent Archival Shadow: Though they returned to their ancestral lands, the photographs, anthropometric measurements, and cinematic reels captured in St. Louis remained trapped in Western institutions, cementing a reductive global caricature that descendants would spend generations working to dismantle and correct.

Ultimately, the physical return to the Cordillera marked the end of their journey across the global exhibition circuit, but it initiated a quiet, generational resistance—one rooted in reclaiming historical truth, preserving indigenous autonomy, and ensuring that the dignity of their communities outlived the transient spectacle of the White City.

Chapter 3

Ota Benga and the Bronx Zoo

The Transition from the World's Fair to the Urban Menagerie

The structural mechanics of human display that were perfected on a massive, industrial scale at the 1904 St. Louis World's Fair did not dissolve with the closing of the exposition. Instead, they contracted, finding new life within the institutional architecture of America's urban centers. If the Louisiana Purchase Exposition served as the grand, national theater for imperial ideology, the events of September 1906 at the New York Zoological Park—commonly known as the Bronx Zoo—represented its most chillingly intimate and concentrated manifestation.

The man at the center of this tragedy was Ota Benga, a young Mbuti man from the Congo Free State. Benga's journey to the United States was brokered by Samuel Phillips Verner, a southern missionary, self-styled explorer, and anthropological collector operating in the Congo under the brutal colonial regime of King Leopold II. Verner had previously acquired individuals to display at the St. Louis fair and was seeking renewed financial backing and academic prestige. Having encountered Benga—whose wife and children had already been murdered by the Force Publique, the colonial military police of the Congo Free State—Verner brought him to the United States, initially presenting him as a living curiosity before arranging his placement at the Bronx Zoo.

The Architecture of Confinement: The Primate House Exhibition

In September 1906, Bronx Zoo Director William Hornaday—a passionate zoologist and conservationist—made the fateful decision to authorize an exhibition that collapsed the boundary between human beings and non-human primates. Benga was assigned a living space within the zoo's Monkey House, sharing quarters with an orangutan named Dohong.

The staging of the exhibit was calculated to invoke evolutionary hierarchy and secure maximum public spectacle:

The Display of the "Missing Link": Zoo signage identified Benga by name, age, origin, and the provocative designation that he was a representative of a "pygmy" race, explicitly framed as an evolutionary steppingstone between apes and civilized humanity.

Props and Performance: To enhance sensationalism, Benga was provided with a bow and arrow, a target to shoot at, and traditional clothing. Visitors were encouraged to watch him perform daily routines, turning his forced captivity into a sideshow attraction.

The Turnout and the Crowd: The public reaction was immediate and overwhelming. Up to forty thousand visitors a day flooded the zoo, crowding around the primate enclosure. The psychological impact on Benga—isolated by language, traumatized by the recent loss of his family in Congo, and caged alongside animals—was profound and immediate.

The Role of Scientific Racism and Institutional Justification

The decision by zoo authorities and affiliated scientists to exhibit Benga was not an isolated aberration; it was deeply rooted in the prevailing intellectual framework of scientific racism that dominated turn-of-the-century American institutions.

Prominent figures within the American Museum of Natural History and the New York Zoological Society operated under unilinear evolutionary assumptions, believing that non-white indigenous populations represented arrested stages of human development. Director William Hornaday and Madison Grant—a prominent eugenicist, zoologist, and co-founder of the New York Zoological Society—defended the exhibition as an educational and scientific endeavor. To them, displaying Benga was a legitimate public demonstration of evolutionary theory, aligning biological science with the broader ideological imperatives of Western racial supremacy and colonial domination.

The Clerical Resistance and Public Controversy

Unlike the Philippine Reservation in St. Louis, which enjoyed public approval and federal protection, the exhibition of Ota Benga sparked immediate, fierce moral outrage led by a coalition of African American clergymen and community leaders in New York.

The Voice of the Black Church: Prominent ministers, most notably Reverend James H. Gordon, superintendent of the Howard Colored Orphan Asylum in Brooklyn, recognized the exhibition for what it was: a grotesque violation of human dignity and a direct assault on the moral standing of people of color in America.

The Mobilization of Protest: The clergy organized immediate protests, petitioning city officials, confronting zoo administration, and generating a wave of critical press coverage that challenged the racial justifications put forth by Hornaday and Grant. They argued that displaying a human being in a zoo degradation not only Benga himself, but all people of African descent by weaponizing science to validate white supremacy.

The Closure of the Exhibit and Benga's Subsequent Fate

Faced with mounting public pressure, escalating legal threats, and intense negative publicity, zoo administrators were forced to dismantle the exhibit within weeks of its opening.

Removal from the Zoo: In late September 1906, Benga was removed from the Monkey House and placed under the care of

Reverend Gordon, who transferred him to the Howard Colored Orphan Asylum.

Subsequent Life and Displacement: Although removed from immediate public cages, Benga remained caught between two worlds. He was placed in a Virginia seminary school to assimilate him into American society, and he learned to speak English and dress in Western attire. However, the outbreak of World War I in 1914 cut off his hopes of returning home to Congo. Deeply homesick and suffering from the accumulated trauma of his displacement, Benga tragically took his own life in March 1916.

The 1906 Bronx Zoo exhibition of Ota Benga stands as a stark reminder of the human cost of scientific racism and the institutionalized cruelty of the human exhibition era. It exposed the dark underbelly of turn-of-the-century progressivism, demonstrating how science and popular entertainment could be weaponized to dehumanize the vulnerable for the amusement of empire.

The Early Life of Ota Benga: Origins, Family, and the Shadow of the Congo Free State

To fully grasp the magnitude of the tragedy that unfolded at the Bronx Zoo in September 1906, one must look beyond the gates of the New York Zoological Park and examine the world from which Ota Benga was forcibly uprooted. Born around 1883 in the equatorial rainforests of the Congo basin, Benga was a member of the Mbuti people, a forest-dwelling group traditionally inhabiting the region surrounding the Kasai River. His early life was defined by the deep, intricate cultural traditions of his community: a nomadic, foraging lifestyle rooted in a profound ecological harmony with the rainforest, communal social structures, and a rich oral history passed down through generations.

However, the world of Benga's youth was violently upended by one of the most brutal imperial regimes in human history: the Congo Free State, administered as the personal, private property of King Leopold II of Belgium. Under Leopold's rule, the region was subjected to a systematic reign of terror driven by the global rubber boom. Armed colonial militias—most notably the Force Publique—enforced draconian rubber-gathering quotas through horrific acts of mass mutilation, hostage-taking, and indiscriminate slaughter.

It was within this crucible of state-sponsored violence that Benga's life was shattered. In a brutal raid by the Force Publique on his village, Benga's camp was destroyed, and his wife and two children were murdered. Benga himself was captured, surviving only because he had been away hunting in the deep forest when the raid occurred. This catastrophic trauma left him isolated and vulnerable, setting the stage for his encounter with Samuel Phillips Vcrncr—an Amcrican missionary, sclf-styled explorer, and collector operating in the Congo under the guise of scientific inquiry. Verner, capitalizing on the chaos and devastation wrought by Leopold's regime, acquired Benga—along with several other Congolese individuals—to fulfill commissions for American museums and exposition organizers, tearing him away from his ancestral homeland and ferrying him across the Atlantic toward an entirely alien and hostile world.

The Encounter with Verner and the Transatlantic Crossing

The fateful intersection between Ota Benga and Samuel Phillips Verner in 1904 marked the definitive severing of Benga's ties to the Congo basin and initiated his transition into a globally commodified specimen. Verner, operating with financial backing from the Louisiana Purchase Exposition Commission and academic interests such as the Smithsonian Institution, was scouring the interior of the Congo Free State for human exhibits to populate the upcoming St. Louis World's Fair.

The Transaction of Captivity: Vulnerable, grieving the violent loss of his family, and surviving as a displaced refugee within a war-torn landscape, Benga was in no position to offer informed autonomous consent. Verner secured Benga—alongside several other Congolese youths and men—through a mixture of financial negotiation with local intermediaries, promises of safe return, and the sheer coercive leverage of a regime where European authority held absolute life-and-death power.

The Voyage Across the Atlantic: Stripped of his community, his language, and his familiar forest environment, Benga was thrust onto a steamship bound for North America. The transatlantic crossing marked his introduction to the modern industrial machinery of the West. Confined below deck alongside cargo and expedition equipment, Benga experienced firsthand the displacement that characterized the global reach of turn-of-the-century imperialism.

The St. Louis Prelude: Upon arriving in the United States, Benga and his companions were initially displayed at the 1904 St. Louis World's Fair as part of the anthropology exhibits managed by William John McGee. Though less documented in mainstream public records than the Philippine Reservation, Benga was subjected to the same invasive anthropometric measurements, public voyeurism, and pseudoscientific categorization designed to frame him as an evolutionary curiosity. When the fair concluded, Verner returned Benga to Africa temporarily, but the brief repatriation proved hollow; rootless, and with his home village destroyed, Benga willingly or under renewed persuasion accompanied Verner back to the United States in 1906, ultimately walking directly into the trap of the Bronx Zoo.

The Aftermath and Legacy of Ota Benga

Following the closure of the Bronx Zoo exhibition in September 1906, Ota Benga's life became a permanent struggle to reclaim his autonomy amidst the wreckage of paternalistic exploitation. Transferred to the custody of Reverend James H. Gordon, Benga was placed in the Howard Colored Orphan Asylum in Brooklyn, where well-meaning reformers attempted to assimilate him into American society. He was taught to speak English, dressed in Western clothing, and later relocated to Lynchburg, Virginia, to distance him from the relentless media circus of New York.

In Virginia, Benga found brief moments of peace among local African American families, working at a tobacco factory and even discarding his traditional filed teeth to blend in. However, the profound psychological trauma of his displacement—compounded by the outbreak of World War I in 1914, which permanently shattered any remaining hope of returning to his surviving family or homeland in the Congo—proved insurmountable. Deeply homesick and overwhelmed by depression, Ota Benga tragically took his own life on March 20, 1916.

The tragic end of Benga's life left an indelible stain on the American scientific and cultural institutions that had treated his humanity as a commodity. The episode forced a rare, albeit fleeting, public reckoning regarding the ethical boundaries of scientific inquiry, racial display, and the dark realities of exhibition culture at the height of the imperial era. Today, historians, descendants, and cultural advocates continue to honor Benga's memory—ensuring that his true story as a resilient human being stolen by empire is never again overshadowed by the cruel spectacle of the primate house.

The Long Shadow and Institutional Reckoning

More than a century after Ota Benga was caged within the primate house of the Bronx Zoo, the deep historical wounds inflicted by his exploitation have prompted formal institutional reckonings. In July 2020, over a century after the tragic event, the Wildlife Conservation Society—the organization operating the Bronx Zoo—issued a comprehensive and long-overdue formal apology. Leadership publicly condemned the "disgraceful" treatment of

Benga and acknowledged the institution's historical complicity in promoting scientific racism and white supremacy.

Simultaneously, historical preservation efforts in Lynchburg, Virginia—where Benga spent his final years and found temporary sanctuary among local community members and poets like Anne Spencer—have worked to restore his dignity. Memorial markers and annual remembrance ceremonies now stand to honor his memory, ensuring that his identity as a resilient human being stolen by empire is preserved.

Through these modern acts of truth-telling and archival transparency, endures not merely as a chronicle of cruelty, but as a permanent reminder of the enduring human capacity to demand justice, reclaim stolen histories, and confront the darkest chapters of the past.

114 years after putting an African man on display in its Monkey House, zoo issues apology. Journalist Pamela Newkirk on the tragic history of Ota Benga and the long-overdue institutional apology issued by the Bronx Zoo's operating organization.

The Symbiosis of Print Media and Popular Voyeurism

The rapid escalation of the Ota Benga exhibition from a localized administrative decision to an international scandal was fueled directly by the yellow journalism of the era. Metropolitan newspapers, competing fiercely for circulation numbers, seized upon the presence of a Congolese man in the Primate House with sensational headlines.

The Fabrication of Consent: Journalists and zoo publicists routinely manufactured narratives claiming that Benga was entirely willing, even delighted, to be caged alongside non-human primates. These reports frequently invoked paternalistic tropes, framing the exhibition as a benevolent or educational intervention designed to satisfy public curiosity about human evolution.

The Amplification of Spectacle: Daily tabloids published exaggerated descriptions of Benga's physical appearance, his diet, and his interactions with the orangutan Dohong. This relentless media coverage transformed the zoo into a massive commercial draw, pulling tens of thousands of visitors through the turnstiles daily and embedding racist pseudo-evolutionary theories into the everyday visual culture of urban Americans.

The Ideological Architecture: William Hornaday, Madison Grant, and Scientific Racism

The intellectual scaffolding that permitted the caging of a human being in a zoological park was erected by leading figures of the American scientific establishment. Chief among them was William Hornaday, the founding director of the Bronx Zoo, whose fierce dedication to wildlife conservation was paradoxically matched by a rigid adherence to hierarchical racial taxonomies.

The Influence of Madison Grant: Hornaday worked in close alignment with figures like Madison Grant, a powerful eugenicist, conservationist, and trustee of the New York Zoological Society. Grant's worldview divided humanity into strict, unchangeable racial categories, placing Nordic peoples at the pinnacle of civilization and positioning indigenous African populations near non-human primates.

The Perversion of Evolutionary Science: Under this ideological framework, Primate House was consciously utilized as a living laboratory to demonstrate unilinear social evolution to the general public. To Hornaday, Grant, and their contemporaries, displaying Benga alongside an ape was not an act of cruelty, but a literal, physical manifestation of scientific progress—a living diagram of humanity's supposed evolutionary ascent.

The Intersectional Resistance: Black Clergy and Community Mobilization

While mainstream white newspapers and scientific elites defended or trivialized the exhibit, a powerful and immediate countermovement arose from New York's African American community, led primarily by a coalition of influential clergymen and institutional leaders.

Moral Condemnation and Civil Rights: Prominent figures such as Reverend James H. Gordon recognized that the exhibition was an assault not only on Benga's individual humanity, but on the dignity and civil standing of all people of African descent living in a country marked by rising racial hostility, Jim Crow disenfranchisement, and widespread lynching.

Confronting City Hall and Zoo Management: The clergy organized swift delegations, flooded municipal offices with letters of protest, and threatened legal action against the New York Zoological Society. Their fearless public opposition shattered the consensus of indifference maintained by city officials and forced zoo administrators into a defensive retreat, proving that marginalized communities possessed the moral authority and organizational capacity to challenge institutionalized racism at its core.

The Geopolitical and Colonial Context: King Leopold's Shadow

The tragedy of Ota Benga cannot be fully comprehended without tracing the transnational pathways of colonial violence that delivered him to the United States. His life was shattered by the atrocities committed in the Congo Free State under the personal, corporate tyranny of King Leopold II.

The Destruction of Indigenous Ecosystems: The extraction of rubber and ivory under Leopold's regime relied on systematic terror, forced labor, and mass murder by the Force Publique. Entire communities were decimated, and survivors were left displaced, traumatized, and vulnerable to exploitation by predatory Western collectors like Samuel Phillips Verner.

The Commodification of Trauma: Verner exploited this catastrophic human suffering, weaponizing his position as a white Western explorer to acquire human subjects under the guise of scientific collection. The transition of Benga from a grieving forest-dweller in the Kasai basin to a captive specimen in a New York zoological cage illustrates the seamless pipeline connecting European imperial extraction in Africa to domestic racial spectacles in the United States.

The Long-Term Cultural Impact and Historical Memory

The abrupt closure of the Bronx Zoo exhibition in late September 1906 did not dismantle the structural racism that enabled it, but it marked a critical turning point in the history of human exhibition in America. Following the widespread public backlash and international embarrassment surrounding the Ota Benga controversy, major American institutions largely abandoned the explicit public display of living human beings in zoos and circuses, recognizing the severe reputational and legal risks involved.

However, the cultural legacy of the event persisted beneath the surface, reinforcing paternalistic attitudes that would influence immigration policies, educational curricula, and popular media for generations. It is only in recent decades—through exhaustive archival research, historical reclamation projects, and formal institutional apologies, such as the 2020 statement by the Wildlife Conservation Society—that Ota Benga's true history has been brought to light. By stripping away the layer of protective mythmaking constructed by his captors and zoo administrators, modern scholarship restores Benga's humanity, ensuring that his life, suffering, and quiet resilience remain a permanent testament against the historical crimes of scientific racism and imperial exploitation.

The Final Years in Lynchburg: Sanctuary, Disillusionment, and the Tragedy of Exile

Following his departure from New York and his brief tenure under the care of Reverend James H. Gordon at the Howard Colored Orphan Asylum, Ota Benga was relocated in 1910 to Lynchburg, Virginia. This move was intended to provide him with a quieter environment away from the relentless media scrutiny and hostile gaze of the northern urban centers. In Lynchburg, Benga found a measure of sanctuary and routine within a welcoming local African American community, particularly among prominent residents who offered him housing, companionship, and employment.

Integration and Daily Life in Virginia

Work and Independence: Benga found employment at a local tobacco processing factory, where his physical strength, skill, and industriousness earned him the respect of his co-workers. For a time, he lived a relatively independent life, earning his own wages and moving freely through the community.

Cultural Adaptation: Seeking to blend into his new surroundings and escape the constant reminder of his captivity, Benga made the poignant decision to break the sharp points of his teeth—modifications that had been performed in his youth according to Mbuti custom, but which had been relentlessly weaponized by sensationalist newspapers in New York to paint him as a savage. He also learned English, adopted Western clothing, and formed deep bonds with local children, who were often fascinated by his mastery of forest lore, tracking, and wilderness survival.

The Friendship with Anne Spencer: Among his most significant acquaintances in Lynchburg was the renowned Harlem Renaissance poet Anne Spencer and her husband Edward. Spencer provided Benga with a space of intellectual warmth and deep empathy, recognizing his sharp intelligence, quiet dignity, and the profound, unhealed trauma of his displacement.

The Gathering Storm of World War I

Despite these moments of community and integration, Benga remained haunted by a deep, inescapable sense of homesickness. Throughout his years in Virginia, he frequently expressed an intense desire to return to his homeland in the equatorial rainforests of the Congo basin—to walk among his people, speak his native tongue, and reclaim the life that had been violently stolen from him by King Leopold's regime and predatory American collectors.

By 1914, however, those remaining hopes were completely shattered. The outbreak of the First World War severed maritime trade routes across the Atlantic, making passenger and cargo travel between the United States and the African continent virtually impossible. The global conflict closed the final, narrow door that might have allowed Benga to journey home.

The Tragic Conclusion

As the war dragged on and the realization set in that he would never see the Congo basin again, Benga sank into a profound, insurmountable depression. The accumulated weight of his losses—the murder of his family by the Force Publique, his abduction across the Atlantic, his degrading public exhibition in the St. Louis World's Fair and the Bronx Zoo, and his permanent exile in America—became too heavy a burden to bear.

On the evening of March 20, 1916, behind a tobacco barn in Lynchburg, Ota Benga kindled a small ceremonial fire, removed the caps from his teeth, and, utilizing a borrowed pistol, took his own life. He was approximately thirty-three years old.

His death marked a tragic final chapter in an extraordinary and harrowing life, leaving behind a haunting indictment of the racial cruelty, scientific arrogance, and imperial exploitation that defined turn-of-the-century America.

The Memorialization and Continuing Legacy of Ota Benga

The tragic death of Ota Benga in March 1916 did not immediately yield a public reckoning; instead, local newspapers in Lynchburg published brief, detached notices that framed his suicide through the patronizing lens of homesickness, failing to implicate the systemic forces of imperialism and racism that had driven him to despair. For decades, his story slipped into the shadows of American historical memory, preserved primarily in local folklore and specialized academic texts. However, as the twentieth century gave way to the twenty-first, a concerted effort by historians, biographers, and civil rights advocates brought his harrowing life back into the national and international spotlight.

The Work of Historical Reclamation

Biographical Restoration: Pioneering works, most notably investigative journalist Pamela Newkirk's definitive biography Spectacle: The Astonishing Life of Ota Benga, meticulously reconstructed his life from archival fragments, dismantling the myths propagated by his captors and zoo administrators. These historical accounts restored his identity, emphasizing that he was not a passive specimen, but a resilient individual who fought to retain his dignity under unimaginable oppression.

Educational and Institutional Reckoning: The resurgence of public interest catalyzed a profound reassessment of how museums, zoos, and academic institutions address their complicity in scientific racism. When the Wildlife Conservation Society issued its historic 2020 apology for the Bronx Zoo exhibition, it marked a vital turning point, signaling that major cultural institutions could no longer hide behind historical relativism.

The Living Memory: Today, Ota Benga's legacy endures as a powerful cautionary tale against the dehumanization of marginalized peoples. From memorial markers in Lynchburg to educational curricula worldwide, his story serves as a permanent reminder of the ethical boundaries of science, the enduring cost of empire, and the moral imperative of historical truth.

The Global Resonance: Ota Benga and the Decolonization of Modern Archives

The historical trajectory of Ota Benga's life and tragic death has become a cornerstone in the broader, ongoing global movement to decolonize museums, archives, and scientific institutions. Beyond the specific apologies issued by organizations like the Wildlife Conservation Society, Benga's narrative has forced a fundamental re-evaluation of how cultural heritage, human remains, and historical artifacts are cataloged, interpreted, and displayed across the Western world.

Transforming Archival Practice:

The Ethics of Photographic and Anthropometric Collections: Major research libraries and natural history museums are increasingly auditing their historical holdings—specifically nineteenth and early twentieth-century photographic plates and anthropometric records—to reckon with the non-consensual manner in which they were gathered. Scholars are working to restore the true identities of individuals who were photographed or measured under duress, shifting the archival gaze from objectifying scrutiny to respectful historical recognition.

Challenging Institutional Neutrality: Benga's exploitation by prominent scientists like William Hornaday and Madison Grant exposed the myth of absolute scientific objectivity. Contemporary academic institutions now utilize the Ota Benga case study in ethics curricula to teach students how racial ideologies and political pressures can corrupt scientific inquiry.

The Continuing Duty of Historical Truth-Telling

As descendants of the Mbuti people and global civil rights advocates continue to champion historical transparency, the memory of Ota Benga stands as an unyielding challenge to historical amnesia. His story demands that modern societies look unblinkingly at the dark intersection of science, popular entertainment, and imperial violence—ensuring that the lessons of his suffering inform a more just, empathetic, and accountable future.

The Broader Historiographical Shift: Rewriting the Narrative of the Gilded Age

The sustained academic and public focus on Ota Benga has catalyzed a much larger historiographical reassessment of the American Gilded Age and the Progressive Era. For generations, standard historical narratives celebrated turn-of-the-century America as a period of unprecedented industrial expansion, technological innovation, and democratic maturation. However, the integration of Benga's life story—alongside the histories of the Philippine Reservation and other human exhibits—has forced historians to confront the deep contradictions of the era.

Unmasking the Darker Side of Progressivism

The Paradox of Reform: Many of the prominent figures who championed social reforms, labor rights, and environmental conservation during the early twentieth century simultaneously embraced virulent racial hierarchies and eugenics. Figures like William Hornaday and Madison Grant viewed wildlife conservation and racial engineering as complementary facets of a broader project to protect and elevate Western civilization.

Popular Entertainment as Imperial Propaganda: The mass-market appeal of human exhibitions demonstrates how deeply imperialist and racist ideologies permeated everyday leisure culture. Going to the zoo or visiting a world's fair was not a neutral recreational activity, but an active ritual of citizenship that reinforced white supremacy and justified overseas colonial expansion to the American public.

The Pedagogical Transformation

Today, the integration of Ota Benga's history into high school and university curricula marks a vital shift in how modern education addresses structural racism. By moving away from sanitized versions of history, educators utilize Benga's biography to teach critical media literacy, ethical responsibility in science, and the importance of amplifying marginalized voices. This pedagogical shift ensures that future generations understand how easily institutional power can be weaponized against the vulnerable—and why vigilance, empathy, and historical truth remain essential defenses against injustice.

The Modern Echo: Ota Benga and the Ethics of Digital and Institutional Display Today

While the physical cages of the turn-of-the-century zoological parks and world's fairs have long been dismantled, the core ethical questions raised by the life and death of Ota Benga remain sharply relevant in the contemporary digital and institutional landscape. The mechanisms that allowed a human being to be commodified, digitized into historical archives without consent, and sensationalized for public consumption have evolved, finding new expressions in the twenty-first century.

1. The Digital Panopticon and the Ethics of Archival Display

Today, the commodification of human suffering and indigenous identity has largely transitioned from physical exhibitions to digital spaces.

The Re-traumatization of Historical Media: Historic photographs, anthropological films, and audio recordings of marginalized individuals—often gathered under coercive colonial conditions—are routinely uploaded to online platforms, social media, and digital archives without consent, context, or ethical oversight.

The Modern Spectacle: Much like the yellow journalism and crowds of the Bronx Zoo, viral digital culture frequently strips indigenous and historically marginalized people of their agency, reducing complex human lives to sensationalized clickbait or abstract historical curiosities for online audiences.

2. Institutional Complicity in Science, Tech, and Artificial Intelligence

The ideological framework that justified Ota Benga's display—scientific racism and the belief that certain populations are inherently "other" or sub-human—has experienced alarming modern echoes within technology and data science.

Algorithmic Bias and Surveillance: Contemporary scholarship on artificial intelligence and facial recognition technology frequently draws parallels to historical anthropometry.

Studies have shown how biased datasets, flawed biometric algorithms, and invasive surveillance technologies disproportionately target, misidentify, or dehumanize communities of color, echoing the pseudoscientific categorization championed by figures like Madison Grant and William Hornaday.

The Demand for Ethical Governance: Just as the Bronx Zoo controversy forced a reckoning over the moral boundaries of public institutions, modern technologists, ethicists, and civil rights advocates are locked in a struggle to regulate AI and data collection, ensuring that human dignity is not sacrificed on the altar of technological "progress."

3. The Ongoing Imperative of Decolonization

Ultimately, making Ota Benga's story relevant today means recognizing that the structures of imperialism, institutional indifference, and racial hierarchy did not vanish with the Gilded Age. They were absorbed into modern systems of education, governance, and global media.

By continuing to tell his story with unflinching honesty, modern society acknowledges a vital truth: the safeguarding of human dignity requires constant vigilance against the temptation to view any human life as a spectacle, a statistic, or a commodity. Ota Benga's legacy stands as a timeless, urgent reminder that true progress is measured not by technological innovation alone, but by a society's unwavering commitment to justice, empathy, and the absolute equality of all human beings.

The Enduring Burden of Representation: Ota Benga and the Modern Arts

The profound resonance of Ota Benga's life has extended far beyond historical texts and institutional policy changes, inspiring a vibrant wave of artistic, literary, and musical expression. Contemporary creators have taken up the mantle of memory, using poetry, drama, and visual art to restore Benga's voice and interrogate the enduring legacy of colonial exploitation.

1. Poetry and Literary Reimaginings

For decades, poets and writers have turned to Benga's biography to explore themes of displacement, grief, and survival.

The Work of Literary Recovery: Writers like Carrie Allen McCray—whose mother was friends with Anne Spencer in Lynchburg—wrote deeply moving biographies and poetic tributes that rescued Benga from the one-dimensional caricature constructed by 1906 tabloid newspapers. These works emphasize his interiority, his deep connection to the rainforest, and the excruciating psychological weight of living as a permanent exile.

The Poetic Gaze: In contemporary verse, poets frequently contrast the clinical, voyeuristic gaze of the white scientific establishment with Benga's own internal landscape, subverting the dynamic historical power and returning dignity to his memory.

2. Visual Arts, Performance, and Theater

The theatrical and visual arts have similarly embraced Benga's story as a vital medium for public confrontation and healing.

Dramatizing the Gilded Age: Playwrights and multimedia artists have staged theatrical productions that place the audience directly in the uncomfortable position of the 1906 Bronx Zoo spectators, forcing modern viewers to examine their own complicity in voyeurism and the consumption of marginalized bodies.

Exhibitions and Installation Art: Contemporary artists working in museums incorporate historical artifacts, archival photographs, and indigenous perspectives to critique how institutions have historically curated "otherness." These installations challenge galleries to transform from passive display cases into active sites of truth-telling and restorative justice.

Through these creative endeavors, Ota Benga's story transcends the boundaries of a tragic 2006 or 1906 historical footnote. It becomes a living, breathing dialogue about how society remembers, how art heals, and how culture can actively dismantle the lingering architectures of racism and imperial hubris.

The Unbroken Thread — Conclusion

The tragedy of Ota Benga cannot be safely quarantined within the sepia-toned photographs of 1906 or dismissed as an aberration of a bygone, unenlightened era. His life—from the pristine equatorial rainforests of the Kasai basin to the brutal rubber terror of King Leopold's Congo Free State, across the Atlantic into the stifling cages of the St. Louis World's Fair and the Bronx Zoo, and finally to his poignant sanctuary and desperate end in Lynchburg, Virginia—stands as an enduring monument to the resilience of the human spirit under the most monstrous weights of empire and scientific arrogance.

When we look at Ota Benga today, we are forced to look at ourselves. We confront the uncomfortable reality that the mechanisms which commodified his humanity—sensationalized media, pseudoscientific racism, institutional indifference, and the insatiable appetite for human spectacle—did not vanish with the Gilded Age; they merely mutated. They echo in the digital exploitation of marginalized lives, the biases woven into modern technologies, and the persistent inequalities that shape our global institutions.

Yet, his story is equally a testament to the power of resistance and moral awakening. From the Black clergymen of New York who risked their standing to demand his release, to the poets and historians who fought to rescue his name from oblivion, and the modern institutions forced to reckon with their own dark origins, Ota Benga's legacy compels us toward accountability.

He was never a specimen. He was a son, a hunter, a survivor, and a human being whose dignity no cage could ultimately confine. His memory remains an unyielding challenge. A permanent reminder that history is not merely a record of what was done, but an urgent call for how we must choose to live, see, and honor one another now and in the future.

Chapter 4

Science Without Compassion

The Weaponization of Authority

At the turn of the twentieth century, Western scientific establishments operated with an aura of infallible objectivity. Anthropology, physical anthropology, and emerging biometric methodologies were heralded as the ultimate arbiters of human progress. However, far from being neutral disciplines, these fields served as the ideological architects of imperialism, constructing elaborate racial taxonomies designed to validate European and American global dominance. By wrapping prejudice in the respectable language of science, researchers and institutional leaders legitimized the dehumanization of indigenous peoples worldwide, transforming human beings into mere data points and zoological specimens.

The Rise of Physical Anthropology and Anthropometry

During the late nineteenth and early twentieth centuries, physical anthropology became heavily preoccupied with the physical measurement of the human body practice known as anthropometry. Pioneered by figures influenced by social Darwinism, this pseudo-scientific approach sought to establish a hierarchical ranking of human races based on anatomical metrics.

Measuring the "Other": Anthropologists and curators traveled with colonial expeditions or established stations at international expositions to measure cranial capacities, facial angles, limb proportions, and body densities. These measurements were never gathered for objective comparison; rather, they were deliberately interpreted through a pre-existing lens that viewed white European and American bodies as the peak of human evolution.

The Fallacy of Biological Determinism: Practitioners of anthropometry argued that physical traits directly correlated with intellectual capacity, moral development, and civilizational potential. Indigenous peoples from Africa, Asia, and the Americas were systematically categorized as "primitive" or "child-like," locking them into fixed developmental stages that supposedly justified paternalistic control and colonial subjugation.

The Complicity of Academic Institutions

The legitimacy granted to human exhibitions—such as the displays of Ota Benga and the Philippine Reservation at world's fairs—depended heavily on the active participation of major academic and scientific institutions. Museums, zoological societies, and university departments were not passive observers of these spectacles; they were active organizers and beneficiaries.

The Smithsonian and Museum Networks: Leading scientific organizations provided academic credentials to expeditions scouring the globe for human subjects. By framing these displays as "educational" or "ethnological research," institutions shielded themselves from moral criticism, assuring the public that placing humans on exhibition served a higher scientific purpose.

The Distortion of Evolutionary Theory: Evolutionary science was weaponized to promote unilinear cultural evolution—the false belief that all human societies must pass through identical stages of development, ranging from "savagery" to "civilization." Under this framework, placing a Congolese forest-dweller next to a chimpanzee, as occurred at the Bronx Zoo, was defended by museum directors as a visual demonstration of biological history.

Scientific Authority as a Shield for Cruelty

When public outcry or moral objections arose against the degrading treatment of human exhibits, the perpetrators routinely hid behind the shield of scientific authority.

Dismissing Humanitarian Concerns: Protesters and religious leaders who condemned the humiliation of human captives were often dismissed by scientific elites as sentimental, uneducated, or ignorant of scientific truth. Administrators argued that public exposure to living specimens advanced anthropological knowledge and public enlightenment, thereby outweighing individual suffering.

Institutional Rationalization: By reducing human beings to biological curiosities, science created a moral vacuum. When empathy was replaced by clinical detachment, cruelty was rebranded as research, and exploitation was masked as progress.

Intellectual architecture underpinning turn-of-the-century human exhibitions relied heavily upon the weaponization of academic disciplines, transforming fields like physical anthropology and anthropometry into instruments of ideological justification. During the late nineteenth and early twentieth centuries, these emerging branches of science were not pursued with detached neutrality; instead, they were aggressively marshaled to validate pre-existing imperial ambitions and racial hierarchies. By clothing prejudice in the prestigious language of empirical research, scientists, university departments, and museum curators provided a veneer of legitimacy to the profound systemic abuses of the Gilded Age and the height of Western imperialism.

At the center of this pseudoscientific enterprise was anthropometry—the systematic measurement of the human body. Researchers influenced by social Darwinism traveled alongside colonial expeditions, setting up measuring stations at international expositions, world's fairs, and zoological parks to record cranial capacities, facial angles, limb proportions, and body densities. These measurements were never gathered for the purpose of objective biological comparison. Rather, they were deliberately interpreted through a rigid, ethnocentric framework that positioned white European and American bodies as the absolute apex of human evolution. Practitioners of this methodology argued that physical metrics correlated directly with intellectual capacity, moral development, and civilizational worth. Consequently, indigenous peoples from Africa, Asia, and the Americas were systematically categorized as biologically "primitive," locking them into fixed developmental rungs that supposedly justified their subjugation, paternalistic control, and public display.

This systemic distortion extended deeply into major cultural and academic institutions, which acted as active collaborators rather than passive observers. Prominent natural history museums, zoological societies, and university anthropology departments provided the institutional credentials and funding required to procure human subjects from colonized regions. By framing these acquisitions and public displays as vital educational endeavors or legitimate ethnological research, institutions shielded themselves from moral scrutiny. When human beings were placed on exhibition—whether within the "ethnological villages" of world's fairs or inside zoological parks like the primate house of the Bronx Zoo—academic elites defended the spectacles to the public as living laboratories of human history. They promoted the pseudoscientific doctrine of unilinear cultural evolution, the false belief that all human societies progressed along a single, immutable track from savagery to civilization, thereby transforming profound human suffering into a visual lesson in social progress.

Furthermore, whenever humanitarian concerns, religious objections, or public outrages surfaced against the degrading treatment of human captives, the perpetrators routinely hid behind the impenetrable shield of scientific authority. Protesters, civil rights advocates, and progressive clergymen who condemned the humiliation of individuals like Ota Benga were dismissively labeled as sentimental, uneducated, or profoundly ignorant of biological and anthropological truths. Museum directors, zoological administrators, and university professors argued that public exposure to living specimens advanced vital scientific knowledge and public enlightenment, contending that this supposed educational gain far outweighed any individual suffering or indignity. By reducing complex human beings to mere biological curiosities, the scientific establishment of the era created a profound moral vacuum. In this clinical environment, empathy was systematically replaced by cold detachment, allowing cruelty to be rebranded as objective research and exploitation to be masked as the inevitable price of human progress.

The reliance on scientific authority during this era extended far beyond the immediate confines of exhibition halls and museum galleries, infiltrating public policy, judicial systems, and educational curricula to construct a totalizing ideology of racial supremacy. Prominent figures within the anthropological community authored widely distributed texts, academic journals, and public lectures that reinforced the notion of inherent racial inequality, providing a pseudo-rational justification for exclusionary immigration policies, legally mandated segregation, and aggressive overseas territorial expansion. By positioning racial hierarchy as an immutable law of nature rather than a social construct born of imperial exploitation, these scientists successfully insulated discriminatory social structures from effective moral critique. Consequently, the general public learned to view the subjugation of indigenous populations not as an injustice to be remedied, but as a scientific inevitability dictated by the unyielding laws of evolutionary biology. This widespread cultural acceptance of biological determinism created an environment where empathy for the colonized was actively suppressed, ensuring that systemic exploitation could continue unchecked under the prestigious banner of scientific advancement.

This pervasive ideological conditioning also deeply infected the medical and psychiatric professions, which eagerly adopted the tools of scientific racism to pathologize the natural reactions of colonized and oppressed peoples. When human exhibits or colonial subjects displayed profound psychological distress, despair, or resistance under the crushing weight of captivity, institutional doctors and researchers frequently reinterpreted these symptoms not as normal responses to severe trauma, but as biological evidence of inherent mental inferiority or emotional stuntedness. By medicalizing the suffering caused by imperial violence, the scientific establishment neatly absolved itself of ethical responsibility, framing the psychological casualties of human exhibition as clinical proof of a primitive mind struggling to comprehend civilized existence. This circular logic allowed anthropologists, physicians, and museum administrators to perpetuate systemic cruelty with absolute impunity, secure in the belief that their actions were supported by the unassailable laws of science and nature.

Moreover, the long-term ramifications of this institutionalized cruelty extended well beyond the immediate victims, creating a toxic cultural legacy that normalized the commodification of human life for generations to come. By consistently presenting indigenous peoples as scientific specimens rather than sovereign human beings, the academic establishment eroded public empathy and cultivated a pervasive social apathy toward imperial violence. Newspapers, popular magazines, and educational textbooks eagerly mirrored the language of physical anthropology, reinforcing the false narrative that Western dominance was an inevitable biological triumph rather than a consequence of military conquest and economic exploitation. This relentless cultural reinforcement ensured that the ideology of scientific racism became deeply embedded in the foundational fabric of modern Western society, leaving behind a profound historical wound that contemporary institutions are only now beginning to honestly confront, investigate, and dismantle.

In examining the institutionalized structures of the period, historians note that the normalization of scientific racism relied heavily on the active complicity of university presses, academic journals, and high-profile scientific societies. These elite networks regularly published unverified, fabricated, and overtly biased studies that purported to prove the intellectual and biological inferiority of non-white populations, thereby creating a self-reinforcing loop of institutional prejudice. University laboratories and medical colleges frequently acquired human remains and cultural artifacts through dubious, coercive colonial channels, treating sacred items and deceased individuals as mere biological specimens rather than human beings deserving of basic respect. This systematic commodification stripped indigenous communities of their dignity while insulating the scientific community from ethical oversight, establishing a dangerous precedent where the pursuit of empirical knowledge was explicitly divorced from fundamental human empathy and moral accountability.

The philosophical and ideological architecture that permitted the weaponization of science during the Gilded Age was fundamentally rooted in a corrupted Enlightenment framework—one that weaponized rationality itself to serve the apparatus of global empire. By divorcing scientific inquiry from moral philosophy, institutions like the American Museum of Natural History, the Smithsonian, and various university anthropology departments established a dangerous precedent: the elevation of empirical data collection above human empathy. In this intellectual climate, the human subject ceased to be viewed as a conscious agent possessing inalienable rights, spiritual depth, and emotional complexity. Instead, individuals like Ota Benga were atomized into bone fragments, biometric measurements, and behavioral reactions, cataloged alongside flora and fauna in an obsessive quest to codify white supremacy as an immutable biological law.

This institutional detachment created an echo chamber of authority that resonated across legislative halls, editorial boards, and public classrooms. When anthropologists published monographs detailing cranial indices or cultural evolutionary stages, politicians cited these works to draft restrictive immigration quotas, justify the violent pacification of overseas territories, and uphold domestic segregation laws. Science, in this capacity, functioned as the ultimate ideological laundering machine. It took raw economic exploitation, land theft, and racial terror, and transmuted them into the clean, objective language of evolutionary necessity. The human exhibitions at world fairs and zoological parks were not merely crude forms of popular entertainment; they were living propaganda installations designed to reinforce this state-sanctioned worldview, inviting everyday citizens to participate in the ritualized degradation of the "other" as an exercise in civic education and national pride.

To dig deeper into the contemporary ramifications of this era is to recognize how deeply these positivist blind spots persist within modern scientific and technological frameworks. The underlying impulse to quantify, categorize, and subjugate human populations through biometric metrics did not vanish with the closure of nineteenth-century exhibition halls. It evolved into the digital surveillance architectures, predictive policing algorithms, and genetic profiling systems of the twenty-first century. When marginalized communities are systematically misidentified by facial recognition software, or when data collection practices replicate historical patterns of non-consensual extraction, society bears witness to the lingering ghost of anthropometry. The historical tragedy of Ota Benga thus remains an urgent, unhealed wound permanent caution that whenever scientific and institutional power operates without a rigorous, unyielding ethical compass, human dignity becomes the first casualty of progress.

When Ota Benga was placed on display at the Bronx Zoo in September 1906, the spectacle immediately sparked a firestorm of media attention, national debate, and international headlines. However, the global and domestic reaction was sharply divided, reflecting the deeply entrenched racial prejudices and ideological fault lines of the era.

1. The Local and National Outrage: The Black Church Leads Resistance

While mainstream white society largely viewed the exhibition through a lens of idle curiosity, African American communities and religious leaders recognized the display as an existential assault on the dignity of all people of color.

The Colored Baptist Ministers Conference: Led by figures like Reverend James H. Gordon, New York's Black clergymen organized immediate, fierce opposition. They recognized that housing a human being in a primate house was a thinly veiled endorsement of radical Darwinism designed to prove that people of African descent occupied a subhuman rung on the evolutionary ladder.

The National Press Response: African American newspapers across the United States published blistering editorials condemning the zoo administration, the city government, and the broader culture that allowed such degradation to occur. They petitioned municipal leaders and demanded Benga's immediate release, framing his captivity as a national moral stain.

2. Mainstream Defense and Institutional Apathy

In stark contrast to the swift condemnation from Black communities, the mainstream white establishment and major journalistic outlets largely defended or minimized the outrage.

The Stance of the New York Times: In an infamous 1906 editorial, the New York Times dismissed the public uproar, asserting that it was "absurd to make moan over the imagined humiliation and degradation Benga is suffering". The editors claimed that pygmies were "very low in the human scale" and argued that placing him in a school would be a form of torture compared to the "educational" environment of the zoo.

The Scientific Justification: Zoological director William Hornaday and influential eugenicist Madison Grant defended the exhibit as a legitimate anthropological demonstration, backed by an indifferent public that flooded the zoo—breaking attendance records with over 40,000 visitors a day—all eager to catch a glimpse of the primate house spectacle.

3. International Echoes and Global Indifference

As word of the exhibition crossed the Atlantic, European newspapers in England and France clamored for photographs and sensationalized details.

The Complicity of Empire: Operating at the absolute height of European colonialism—where millions of indigenous Africans were enduring horrific atrocities in King Leopold II's Congo Free State—the international press largely treated Benga's captivity as an amusing American curiosity rather than a human rights violation.

A Normalized Atrocity: The global reaction mirrored the domestic one: a mixture of sensationalist entertainment for the masses and clinical detachment from scientific elites, confirming that the dehumanization of colonized peoples was a shared, international enterprise backed by the full weight of Western cultural authority.

When the reality of Ota Benga's confinement inside the Bronx Zoo primate house crossed international borders, the global response laid bare the terrifying reach of a scientific establishment entirely devoid of moral empathy. Newspapers across Europe, from London to Paris, eagerly picked up the sensationalized wire reports, treating his captivity not as a moral catastrophe, but as an exotic spectacle that validated the prevailing European colonial project. At a time when millions of Congolese were suffering under the genocidal rubber extraction regimes of King Leopold II, the international press corps viewed Benga's exhibition through the exact same distorted lens of imperial paternalism. To the global public and the scientific societies of the Old World, the American display was not an aberration; it was seen as a logical, highly entertaining public demonstration of ethnological "truth," proving that the subjugation and cataloging of non-white bodies was a shared

Western enterprise backed by the unassailable authority of modern science.

The global scientific community watched the unfolding American controversy not with horror, but with professional solidarity and clinical detachment. European anthropometric societies, colonial administration offices, and natural history institutions routinely exchanged correspondence, methodologies, and human specimens, operating as an interconnected transnational network of scientific racism. When British and continental newspapers reported on the Bronx Zoo exhibition, they frequently cited the authority of prominent American curators and eugenicists like Madison Grant to validate their own domestic policies of colonial subjugation in Africa and Asia. Science, functioning entirely without compassion, had successfully built an international echo chamber where cruelty was reframed as empirical inquiry, and the systematic denial of human dignity was celebrated across borders as the triumph of civilized progress over the so-called savage world.

This transnational network of scientific indifference also permeated the colonial medical corps and administrative offices of European empires, where the psychological and physical devastation wrought upon indigenous populations was consistently reinterpreted through a clinical, pathologizing lens. When colonial subjects resisted forced labor, protested land seizures, or exhibited profound trauma under the brutal extraction economies of the late nineteenth and early twentieth centuries, foreign medical officers and anthropologists routinely diagnosed their suffering not as a rational response to state-sponsored violence, but as inherent neurological or psychological inferiority. By stripping these populations of their emotional complexity and reducing their humanity to measurable biological traits, institutional science provided an unbreakable ideological shield for imperial governance. This shared international framework ensured that whether an indigenous person was exploited in the rubber forests of Congo, measured by anthropometrics' in a European colonial station, or caged in a New York zoological park, the underlying mechanism remained identical: an unyielding system of authority that operated entirely without compassion, sacrificing human dignity on the altar of pseudoscientific progress and unchecked imperial ambition.

Furthermore, this transnational alignment of academic institutions, government bodies, and popular media created an environment where the voices of dissent were systematically drowned out by the thunderous applause of a public conditioned to equate technological and scientific advancement with moral superiority. While a small cadre of Black clergymen, progressive activists, and independent journalists fought valiantly to restore Ota Benga's dignity and secure his release, they found themselves locked in ideological combat against a deeply entrenched global consensus. The scientific establishment of the Western world had successfully weaponized its prestige to normalize the commodification of human life, transforming exploitation into education and cruelty into curiosity. This profound ethical failure exposed the dark underbelly of the modern age chilling reminder that when knowledge is divorced from empathy and authority operates without compassion, society becomes entirely capable of rationalizing the most egregious atrocities under the banner of progress.

Archival reports, contemporary press accounts, and institutional records from late 1906 reveal how deeply entrenched scientific racism shaped public discourse when Ota Benga was exhibited at the Bronx Zoo. Mainstream newspapers, most notably The New York Times, actively collaborated with the scientific establishment to manufacture public consent for the spectacle. Headlines such as "Bushman Shares a Cage with Bronx Park Apes" were paired with editorial commentary assuring readers that scientific authorities had accurately categorized indigenous Africans as "low in the human scale". Rather than treating the imprisonment of a human being as a moral failure, major metropolitan outlets framed the exhibition as a benevolent educational demonstration of evolutionary theory, shielding zoo directors and eugenicists from accountability while tens of thousands of paying spectators flooded the gates daily.

The grim reality faced by Ota Benga was far from an isolated incident; rather, it was a prominent manifestation of a vast, industrialized global phenomenon that spanned continents and decades. During the peak of the human exhibition era—stretching from the late nineteenth century through the mid-twentieth century—millions of visitors across Europe and North America flocked to "ethnological villages," world's fairs, circuses, and zoological parks to view human beings placed on display like wild animals.

The Scale of Global Exhibitions

World's Fairs and Imperial Expositions: Massive international expositions in major capitals—such as Paris, London, Antwerp, Chicago, and St. Louis—routinely constructed artificial "native villages". At the 1889 and 1900 Paris World's Fairs, and later at the massive 1931 Paris Colonial Exhibition, tens of millions of visitors stared at indigenous peoples from Africa, Asia, and the Pacific, who were coerced or contractually bound into living in simulated, primitive conditions.

Tragic Tolls and Captivity: The living conditions inside these exhibitions were frequently lethal. Stripped of adequate shelter, exposed to harsh European climates in traditional or semi-nude attire, and lacking immunity to local diseases, countless human captives fell ill. For instance, during the 1897 International Exposition in Tervuren, Belgium, multiple Congolese individuals died of influenza and pneumonia after being forced to perform outdoors. Similar tragedies occurred across German, British, and American shows where performers succumbed to tuberculosis, pneumonia, and despair.

The Slow Decline and Aftermath

Human zoos did not vanish overnight following the 1906 public outcry over Ota Benga. Instead, they evolved alongside mass entertainment, persisting well into the twentieth century before finally fading away due to shifting geopolitical landscapes, the devastation of the World Wars, and the gradual rise of anti-colonial independence movements. For decades, the human remains and cultural artifacts gathered during these exhibitions remained locked away in Western Museum basements, stripped of individual identities. Only in recent years have European and American institutions begun confronting this dark heritage through formal apologies, archival reckonings, and the repatriation of remains to their descendants.

The global normalization of human exhibitions relied upon a shared transnational architecture of academic complicity, where scientific institutions across borders collaborated to provide intellectual cover for systemic exploitation. When international expositions in Paris, London, Antwerp, and St. Louis constructed elaborate ethnological villages, they did so with the active endorsement of anthropological societies and natural history museums that viewed these living displays as invaluable opportunities for empirical research. Foreign researchers eagerly visited these sites to record measurements, take photographs, and collect ethnographic data, operating under the comfortable delusion that their clinical detachment absolved them of any moral culpability. This cross-border exchange of pseudoscientific methodologies ensured that the degradation of indigenous peoples was never viewed as a localized aberration, but rather as a standardized, internationally validated practice that reinforced the perceived natural order of global white supremacy.

Furthermore, this institutionalized cruelty was seamlessly integrated into the popular consciousness through the sensationalized reporting of international journalism, which consistently echoed the paternalistic rhetoric of the scientific elite. European and American newspapers framed the presence of colonized peoples in zoos and exposition halls not as a human rights crisis, but as an exciting, educational window into the dawn of human history. By reducing complex human beings to exotic curiosities for public entertainment, the media successfully stripped away their individuality and emotional depth, conditioning millions of citizens to view imperial subjugation as a benevolent act of civilizational uplift. This powerful alignment between academic authority, institutional power, and mass media created an impervious ideological fortress, ensuring that any voices of moral outrage or humanitarian concern were effectively silenced by the overwhelming consensus of a society intoxicated by the myth of scientific progress.

During the era when human zoos, world fairs, and colonial exhibitions were at their peak in the late nineteenth and early twentieth centuries, no specific international laws or treaties explicitly banned the public display of human beings.

Because international law at the time was largely formulated by Western imperial powers to regulate state-to-state commerce and warfare—while actively justifying colonialism through the doctrines of racial hierarchy and Social Darwinism—human captives were legally unprotected. The foundational human rights frameworks, oversight bodies, and global conventions we take for granted today simply did not exist.

The Evolution of International Legal Protections

The systemic practices that allowed individuals like Ota Benga to be caged, studied, and commodified were ultimately dismantled not by a sudden single piece of legislation targeting "human zoos," but by the gradual, hard-won establishment of modern international human rights law following the devastation of the twentieth century:

The Universal Declaration of Human Rights (UDHR, 1948): Adopted by the United Nations in the wake of World War II, the UDHR established foundational legal and moral principles explicitly rejecting the degradation of human beings. Article 5 states that "no one shall be subjected to torture or to cruel, inhuman or degrading treatment or punishment."

International Conventions on Discrimination and Indigenous Rights: Subsequent treaties—such as the International Convention on the Elimination of All Forms of Racial Discrimination (1965) and the UN Declaration on the Rights of Indigenous Peoples (UNDRIP)—created binding international standards that outlaw state-sanctioned racial discrimination, cultural exploitation, and the commodification of indigenous bodies and human remains.

Cultural Property and Repatriation Laws: Modern international frameworks, guided by organizations like UNESCO, now govern the ethical handling of human remains and cultural heritage, compelling museums and academic institutions worldwide to repatriate stolen remains and artifacts back to their ancestral communities.

The absence of specific international legal prohibitions during the height of the human exhibition era highlights a profound structural vacuum in global governance. Throughout the late nineteenth and early twentieth centuries, international law was constructed almost exclusively by Western imperial powers to facilitate cross-border commerce, protect sovereign state boundaries, and codify colonial expansion. Within this legal paradigm, human beings from non-Western territories were systematically classified not as legal people possessing inherent rights, but as colonial subjects or biological specimens. Consequently, transnational treaties and agreements contained no mechanisms to prevent natural history museums, zoological gardens, or exposition promoters from capturing, transporting, and publicizing indigenous populations for entertainment and research.

The global shift away from this institutionalized commodification required a complete restructuring of international law in the wake of twentieth-century atrocities. The legal architecture that finally rendered human zoos and ethnological exhibitions legally impossible emerged through several foundational instruments:

The Universal Declaration of Human Rights (1948): Formulated to establish an unassailable global standard of human dignity, the UDHR directly dismantled the philosophical underpinnings of scientific racism. Articles safeguarding the right to liberty, security of person, and protection from cruel, inhuman, or degrading treatment ensured that state-sanctioned public degradation could no longer be legally justified under the guise of scientific education.

International Human Rights Covenants: Binding treaties such as the International Covenant on Civil and Political Rights (ICCPR) translated these moral imperatives into enforceable international law, prohibiting arbitrary detention, degrading treatment, and racial subjugation by state or private actors.

Decolonization and Indigenous Rights Frameworks: Later developments, including the UN Declaration on the Rights of Indigenous Peoples (UNDRIP), established collective legal rights protecting indigenous cultures, human remains, and heritage from forced extraction, exploitation, and non-consensual scientific display.

During the height of the human exhibition era in the late nineteenth and early twentieth centuries, no nation possessed specific domestic or international laws explicitly banning "human zoos" or ethnological expositions. Because the legal and political structures of Western imperial powers—including the United States, Belgium, France, Germany, and the United Kingdom—were thoroughly saturated by the doctrines of scientific racism and colonial expansion, the institutionalized display of indigenous peoples operated entirely within a protected legal vacuum. Rather than being prohibited by statute, these exhibitions were actively facilitated, funded, and authorized by municipal governments and national administrations who viewed them as legitimate instruments of civic education and imperial propaganda.

How major nations handled or failed to regulate these events reveals the depth of institutional complicity across the Western world:

The United States: During Ota Benga's confinement at the Bronx Zoo in 1906, American federal and state laws contained no statutes protecting human captives from public exhibition or degrading treatment. Local authorities and municipal park commissioners actively defended the display, and no criminal charges were ever filed against the zoo administration. Instead, the resolution of the crisis relied entirely on private advocacy, religious protests, and moral pressure led by African American clergymen, which eventually forced the zoo to release Benga into temporary custody.

France: As a primary hub for colonial expositions—such as the massive human displays hosted at the Jardin d'Acclimatation in Paris and the 1931 Paris Colonial Exhibition—French domestic law treated indigenous participants through the framework of colonial administration rather than universal civil rights. Performers from regions like New Caledonia or French West Africa were bound by restrictive contracts overseen by the Ministry of Colonies, possessing zero legal recourse against exploitation, forced exposure to harsh European climates, or non-consensual anthropological measurement.

Belgium: During international exhibitions in Brussels and Tervuren (such as those in 1897 and 1958), the Belgian government directly sponsored "Congolese villages" to generate public support for King Leopold's brutal economic enterprises in the Congo Free State. Belgian laws at the time drew a rigid, absolute line between

Belgian citizens and colonial subjects, denying the latter basic human rights and legal standing, thereby ensuring that the immense suffering and deaths occurring within these exhibitions went entirely unpunished by the courts.

Germany: Imperial and Weimar-era Germany heavily integrated ethnological shows into public zoological gardens, such as Carl Hagenbeck's animal and human exhibitions in Hamburg. Domestic laws governing public entertainment and animal welfare contained zero provisions regarding the ethical treatment of human beings from foreign territories. When these exhibitions declined in the early 1930s, the performers left behind faced severe legal limbo, stripped of citizenship rights and subjected to systemic state-backed discrimination.

Ultimately, because the legal codes of these nations were deliberately structured to uphold racial hierarchies, no domestic legislation existed to dismantle human zoos from within. It required the catastrophic collapse of the European imperial order, the horrors of mid-century total war, and the subsequent establishment of modern international human rights frameworks—such as the 1948 Universal Declaration of Human Rights—to finally outlaw the legal, social, and physical conditions that permitted human beings to be caged and displayed as scientific specimens.

The absence of legal safeguards was not unique to the major Western imperial hubs; it extended globally to other nations that either hosted human exhibitions or participated in the international circuits of ethnological display during the nineteenth and twentieth centuries. Across different political systems, domestic laws consistently failed to protect non-dominant or colonized populations from public commodification because state legal frameworks were explicitly designed to serve nationalist expansion, racial categorization, or assimilation policies.

Japan: During domestic industrial and national expositions—such as the National Industrial Exhibitions and the 1903 Osaka Exposition—Japan displayed indigenous populations, including Ainu from Hokkaido, Okinawans, and Taiwanese aborigines, as well as Koreans. Japanese domestic law at the time contained no prohibitions against human exhibitions. Instead, these displays were organized and sanctioned by government authorities to visually reinforce imperial hierarchies, promote national modernization, and justify colonial expansion across Asia by depicting neighboring groups as "backward" or "primitive".

The German Empire and Weimar Republic: Long before and after losing its overseas colonies, Germany was a primary global center for "anthropological zoological" displays managed by impresarios like Carl Hagenbeck. German public entertainment and administrative laws drew strict legal boundaries based on nationality and race, leaving foreign performers and colonized subjects with zero statutory protection against exploitation, breach of contract, or hazardous living conditions.

The United Kingdom: While domestic laws strictly forbade public exhibitions of a degrading nature for British citizens, those legal protections did not apply to subjects from the British Empire. Imperial subjects brought to London for the Great Exhibitions, the British Empire Exhibition at Wembley, or commercial circuses operated under an entirely separate, exploitative legal status managed by the Colonial Office. These contracts treated human performers as economic assets rather than citizens possessing fundamental labor or civil rights.

In every country that participated in or hosted human fairs, domestic legislation acted as an instrument of state ideology rather than a shield for human rights. Because the global legal consensus viewed non-Western peoples through a lens of racial paternalism, no nation enacted laws to stop human zoos; rather, their legal codes actively facilitated the exhibitions as vital exercises in nationalist pageantry and scientific progress.

The inclusion of the Philippines—specifically the display of indigenous Igorot people at the massive 1904 St. Louis World's Fair (Louisiana Purchase Exposition)—offers a striking illustration of how domestic and colonial laws were manipulated to facilitate human exhibitions. Following the Philippine-American War, the United States government directly financed and orchestrated a sprawling 47-acre Philippine Reservation housing over 1,100 Filipinos across various ethnic groups, with the Igorot village serving as one of the most heavily promoted and sensationalized spectacles.

Examining the legal realities surrounding the Igorot exhibition reveals a complete absence of protective statutes, paired with active state and municipal coordination:

The United States and Insular Frameworks: Under American domestic law at the time, residents of newly acquired territories like the Philippines occupied a legally ambiguous status as "non-citizen nationals," denying them fundamental constitutional protections. Consequently, no federal or state laws prohibited promoters, anthropologists, or government officials from transporting the Igorot people to the U.S. or placing them on public display. Contracts managed by exposition boards treated the performers as economic assets and scientific subjects rather than protected laborers or citizens.

Local Jurisdictional Clashes: The legal vacuum frequently created localized friction, such as when local law enforcement officers in cities hosting traveling spinoff shows—unfamiliar with or indifferent to traditional indigenous attire—arrested performers on grounds of indecent exposure. These sporadic arrests highlighted how municipal legal codes were weaponized against the performers rather than protecting them from exploitation.

The Shift in Legislative Pressure: Unlike earlier exhibitions that operated with absolute impunity, the intense public discomfort, protests by Filipino students and intellectuals in the U.S., and eventual international scandals (such as performers being abandoned destitute in Europe by private showmen like Richard Schneidewind) finally triggered legislative action. By 1914, mounting pressure forced the U.S. government to enact specific legislation in the Philippines strictly forbidding the recruitment and export of indigenous groups for commercial and exhibition purposes, effectively bringing an end to the state-sanctioned trafficking of Igorot performers.

Archival documentation and historical accounts surrounding the 1904 St. Louis World's Fair—and subsequent commercial offshoots managed by rogue impresarios like Truman Hunt at Coney Island—reveal that the exploitation of the Igorot people was meticulously engineered to serve American imperial strategy. The U.S. government, under the guidance of colonial administrators such as William Howard Taft, financed a massive 47-acre Philippine Reservation designed to display over 1,100 indigenous Filipinos across hierarchical "villages". The explicit political objective was to manufacture public consent for overseas colonization by visually arguing that Filipinos were "uncivilized" and entirely unready for self-governance. Central to this propaganda campaign was the sensationalized display of the Igorot people, whose traditional clothing and ceremonial practices—most notably the coerced, daily butchering and consumption of dogs sourced from local pounds—were stripped of their cultural context, sensationalized by the mainstream press, and weaponized to cement racist caricatures of savagery in the American consciousness.

Actions and Responses of the Philippine Government and Leadership

During the initial years of these exhibitions (the early 1900s), the formal legislative and administrative apparatus in the Philippines was entirely under the control of the American colonial government (the Philippine Commission and the Bureau of Insular Affairs). Consequently, local official channels initially facilitated or turned a blind eye to the recruitment and export of indigenous groups. However, as the human toll mounted—marked by broken contracts, severe weather exposure, unpaid wages by independent showmen like Truman Hunt and Richard Schneidewind, and instances of performers being abandoned destitute in foreign cities like Ghent—opposition swelled.

Protests by Filipino Intellectuals and Students: Educated Filipinos, nationalists, and students living or studying abroad vocally condemned the expositions, organizing public resistance and petitioning authorities against the national humiliation and mistreatment of their indigenous compatriots.

Legislative and Administrative Crackdowns: As mounting scandals, public abuses, and humanitarian crises made international news, pressure forced colonial and local authorities to shift policy. By the 1910s, the Philippine Assembly and colonial administration began enacting strict regulatory barriers and executive restrictions. These measures effectively outlawed the recruitment, contracting, and overseas transportation of indigenous Filipinos for commercial exhibitions and human zoos, finally cutting off the supply lines that had allowed impresarios to traffic human beings across international fair circuits.

The systematic exploitation of indigenous peoples within global exhibitions ultimately exposed the profound complicity of transnational scientific networks, which continuously manufactured pseudoscientific justifications to protect imperial ambitions. Whether through the confinement of Ota Benga in New York or the orchestration of the 47-acre Philippine Reservation at the 1904 St. Louis World's Fair, academic elites and government administrators operated hand in hand to transform human dignity into a consumable spectacle. By reducing diverse cultures to static markers of "savagery", these institutional architectures shielded perpetrators from accountability under the guise of educational progress. It required global reckoning, decades of advocacy, and the eventual establishment of modern international human rights frameworks to dismantle the legal and philosophical structures that permitted this widespread human exploitation.

Expanding our understanding of this era requires looking closely at how international academic institutions and anthropological networks formed a tight-knit echo chamber that actively sustained global white supremacy. Across European and American universities, the emerging disciplines of physical anthropology, ethnology, and eugenics were not operating on the fringes of society; they sat at the absolute center of intellectual prestige. When human beings were displayed in zoological parks, world fairs, and colonial expositions, university departments were the first to request access to the captives. Anthropologists utilized craniometry, plaster casting, and exhaustive physiological measurements to turn living, breathing individuals into clinical datasets. This academic validation gave impresarios and municipal governments the moral cover they needed, allowing them to market profound cruelty as cutting-edge science and public enlightenment.

Furthermore, this international defense of dehumanization heavily relied on the circulation of academic journals, global scientific congresses, and transnational museum networks. Scholars from Berlin, Paris, London, and New York regularly corresponded, sharing techniques on how best to classify, photograph, and catalog colonized populations. When critics or humanitarian groups raised objections against the degradation of human captives, the international scientific establishment closed ranks, dismissing ethical concerns as sentimental ignorance that threatened the forward march of human knowledge. This global network ensured that the rationalization of empire was not merely a political project, but an institutionalized intellectual crusade—proving that the most devastating atrocities of the modern era were often championed not by the ignorant, but by the educated elite operating entirely without empathy.

When stripped of the sanitized academic jargon and paternalistic euphemisms invented by nineteenth-century elites, the global phenomenon of human zoos reveals itself for what it truly was: a state-sanctioned, industrialized trade in human trafficking and torture. How else can history define an enterprise where human beings were hunted across continents, locked in cages next to wild animals, stripped of their clothing, forced into sub-zero climates, and dissected by academic sadists under the glowing banner of "progress"? The international scientific establishment did not merely observe these atrocities—they weaponized their authority to institutionalize sadism, transforming the humiliation of Black and Indigenous bodies into a lucrative, globally coordinated spectator sport.

This raises an aggressive, inescapable question for the modern world: why did the architects, financiers, and academic perpetrators of these human exhibitions escape criminal prosecution, financial ruin, and moral damnation? While low-level showmen like Truman Hunt occasionally faced minor blowback, the elite anthropologists, university deans, museum directors, and government ministers who engineered, funded, and profited from this mass dehumanization walked away entirely unpunished. They retired to prestigious academic chairs, received state honors, and left behind legacies still celebrated in university halls.

When institutional power, scientific prestige, and media compliance unite to rationalize cruelty, society loses its moral compass entirely proving that the most barbaric acts in human history are rarely committed by monsters in the shadows, but by respectable, educated men in suits operating in broad daylight.

The historical architecture of human exhibitions stands as an indelible testament to what transpires when institutional power operates completely detached from moral conscience. Across continents, municipal authorities, academic societies, and commercial promoters forged an international consensus that rendered human trafficking and public degradation acceptable under the guise of public education. Yet, the systemic impunity enjoyed by the architects of these displays could not withstand the ultimate evolution of global consciousness. As the horrors of twentieth-century total war forced a fundamental reevaluation of human rights, the intellectual pillars of scientific racism crumbled, exposing the deeply flawed, highly politicized nature of anthropometry and colonial anthropology.

The legacy of this era demands more than passive historical acknowledgment; it requires an active, ongoing interrogation of how institutional bias, data exploitation, and systemic dehumanization manifest in the modern world. From the repatriation of indigenous human remains stored in museum basements to the critical reexamination of modern biometric and surveillance systems, contemporary society continues the unfinished work of dismantling the structures built during the height of the exhibition era. Restoring dignity to those who were commodified, caged, and studied without consent is not merely an exercise in historical correction—it is an essential safeguard to ensure that science and governance never again sacrifice human rights on the altar of unyielding progress.

The true horror of the human exhibition era lies not merely in the acts of confinement themselves, but in the terrifying ease with which intellectual elites normalized atrocity. When university lecture halls, natural history museums, and government offices harmonize to strip fellow human beings of their fundamental rights, the boundary between civilization and barbarism collapses entirely. The legacy of Ota Benga, the Igorot villagers of the 1904 St. Louis World's Fair, and the countless unnamed victims displayed across global fairgrounds serves as an eternal warning against the dangers of institutional apathy.

Today, as cultural institutions slowly grapple with this dark inheritance—returning stolen ancestral remains, rewriting whitewashed historical plaques, and confronting the ghosts of scientific racism—the world is reminded that history is never truly dead. The structures of exploitation may change their outward appearance, trading cage bars for algorithms and public spectacles for covert biometric tracking, but the core temptation remains: the drive to quantify, categorize, and commodify human life for the benefit of the powerful. Refusing to let that legacy repeat requires an unwavering commitment to a singular truth—that human dignity is absolute, non-negotiable, and can never be subordinated to the cold calculations of progress.

On this dark era of global history, society must confront the uncomfortable reality that human zoos and ethnological expositions were not historical anomalies or sudden explosions of madness. They were the logical, highly organized products of an intellectual ecosystem that taught people to look at their fellow human beings not with empathy, but with clinical detachment. When science becomes a tool for domination rather than discovery, and when institutions prioritize prestige over basic humanity, cruelty is easily dressed up as civic progress.

The enduring responsibility of the modern era is to ensure that the voices of those who suffered—from the indigenous peoples exhibited on world stages to the families whose ancestors were treated as museum specimens—are never again silenced by institutional indifference. Recognizing this history is not merely about condemning the past; it is about building a permanent, unbreakable defense for human rights, ensuring that no individual, community, or culture is ever again reduced to a spectacle for the amusement of the powerful.

The ghosts of the exhibition halls—whether haunting the archival records of the Bronx Zoo, the sprawling fairgrounds of St. Louis, or the colonial expositions of Europe—continue to demand an unyielding accounting from history. They remind us that the distance between civilized pretense and profound barbarism is bridged the moment society permits any group of human beings to be measured, categorized, and stripped of their intrinsic worth.

As contemporary generations push to purge the lingering residues of scientific racism from modern institutions, museums, and educational curricula, the lessons of this era remain clear. True progress is measured not by the velocity of technological advancement or the expansion of empirical data, but by how fiercely society protects the dignity, autonomy, and humanity of the most vulnerable. Only by maintaining eternal vigilance against the cold, unfeeling architectures of exploitation can the modern world honor the memory of those who endured the dark machinery of the human exhibition era.

The enduring mandate left by the victims of the human exhibition era is a profound caution for every generation that follows. When the tools of science, law, and media are co-opted to serve systems of oppression, the resulting destruction is measured not just in physical confinement, but in the systematic erasure of human identity.

Ensuring that this history is never repeated requires a steadfast refusal to look away from the uncomfortable truths of our shared past. By holding institutions accountable, challenging modern manifestations of bias, and placing human dignity at the absolute center of ethical inquiry, society can honor the memories of those who were commodified. The ultimate lesson of Chapter 4 remains absolute: knowledge without empathy is tyranny, and progress without humanity is merely cruelty disguised as civilization.

The final measure of any civilization is not found in the grandiosity of its monuments, the reach of its empires, or the volume of its scientific discoveries, but in how it treats its most vulnerable members. The institutionalized cruelty of the human exhibition era stands as a stark reminder of what happens when intellectual arrogance eclipses basic human empathy.

As we look back across the decades that separate the modern world from the crowded fairgrounds of St. Louis, Paris, and New

York, the mandate is clear. We carry a collective responsibility to ensure that the stories of those who were commodified, silenced, and studied without consent are never lost to history. By confronting the uncomfortable truths of scientific racism, holding modern institutions ethically accountable, and fiercely guarding the unalienable dignity of every human being, we ensure that the dark machinery of the past remains forever shuttered, and that progress is never again severed from compassion.

The echoes of the exhibition halls no longer ring with the applause of paying crowds, but their resonance remains deeply embedded in the foundational structures of modern institutions. Every repatriation of a stolen ancestor, every rewriting of a colonial museum plaque, and every critical reexamination of historical archives is a direct challenge to the legacy of scientific racism.

This ongoing reckoning teaches us that history is not a static list of dates and events, but an active dialogue between past injustices and present responsibilities. By keeping the memory of those who suffered alive—and by holding modern science, technology, and governance to the highest ethical standards, society ensures that humanity, empathy, and dignity will forever remain the true measures of progress.

Historical archives, contemporary newspapers, and institutional records reveal a stark polarization in what people said about human zoos and ethnological exhibitions. Public reaction was defined by a fierce collision between mainstream rationalization and sharp, moral condemnation.

The Mainstream Press and General Public: Major metropolitan newspapers and large crowds largely viewed the displays through a lens of entertainment, curiosity, and imperial pride. For example, during the 1906 controversy surrounding Ota Benga's confinement in the Bronx Zoo primate house, The New York Times published an infamous editorial dismissing the public uproar as absurd, claiming that pygmies were "very low in the human scale" and arguing that the zoo offered an "educational" environment. Tens of thousands of paying visitors flooded the turnstiles daily, treating human beings as exotic novelties.

The African American Church and Civil Rights Leaders: In stark contrast, Black religious leaders, community advocates, and minority newspapers expressed profound outrage, recognizing the exhibitions as existential assaults on human dignity. Reverend James H. Gordon, writing on behalf of the Colored Baptist Ministers Conference to New York's mayor, protested sharply: "Our race, we think, is depressed enough without exhibiting one of us with the apes... We think we are worthy of being considered human beings, with souls." Prominent clergymen like Dr. Robert Stuart MacArthur similarly condemned the spectacle in the press, criticizing society for sending missionaries abroad while brutalizing an individual at home.

The Scientific and Academic Establishment: Anthropologists, museum curators, and eugenicists issued reports and statements defending the exhibitions as vital scientific demonstrations. They framed the public display of indigenous peoples as empirical research into human evolution, dismissing ethical protests as uneducated sentimentality that threatened the advancement of science.

The Weight of the Archive

The documentary record left behind by contemporary observers—spanning police reports, municipal permits, missionary logs, and overseas dispatches—provides an unvarnished window into the daily reality of human exhibitions. These reports reveal a system where human beings were routinely tracked, cataloged, and managed just like imported livestock or botanical specimens.

For instance, records from the Louisiana Purchase Exposition Commission in 1904 meticulously detailed the daily food rations, housing logistics, and medical quarantine procedures for the indigenous groups housed on the Philippine Reservation. Bureaucrats and science administrators filed exhaustive reports tracking illness, birth rates, and behavioral compliance among the captives, treating human suffering entirely as logistical data points. Conversely, the archived petitions, frantic telegrams, and scathing resolutions sent by civil rights advocates, concerned clergymen, and foreign diplomats highlight the desperate resistance waged against this institutionalized cruelty. These conflicting documents demonstrate how easily a society can normalize atrocity when administrative efficiency completely replaces moral conscience.

Voices of Resistance: The Advocates Who Fought the Spectacle

While the institutional machinery of the Western scientific establishment and mainstream press largely defended or turned a blind eye to human exhibitions, a courageous vanguard of religious leaders, community advocates, and independent thinkers rose up to challenge the atrocities. These figures risked their reputations and resources to dismantle the systemic normalization of human trafficking and public degradation.

Reverend James H. Gordon: As the supervisor of the Howard Colored Orphan Asylum in Brooklyn and a leading voice in the Colored Baptist Ministers Conference, Reverend Gordon spearheaded the primary domestic resistance against Ota Benga's confinement at the Bronx Zoo in 1906. Mobilizing local clergy and legal threats, Gordon forcefully rebuked zoo administrators, famously declaring to the press and municipal leaders: "Our race, we think, is depressed enough, without exhibiting one of us with the apes. We think we are worthy of being considered human beings, with souls." His persistent advocacy ultimately secured Benga's release from the zoo and provided him with safe sanctuary.

Dr. Robert Stuart MacArthur: A prominent New York City clergyman who acted as a spokesperson for the delegation of Black churches and concerned religious leaders. MacArthur joined forces with Reverend Gordon, petitioning Mayor George B. McClellan Jr. and utilizing his platform to publicly condemn the moral bankruptcy of displaying a human being alongside primates under the guise of scientific education.

Gregory W. Hayes: As the president of the Virginia Theological Seminary and College (now Virginia University of Lynchburg), Hayes became a vital advocate for Ota Benga following his release from New York. Recognizing the psychological toll of the exhibition and the broader assaults of scientific racism, Hayes and his family provided a protective home, education, and community integration for Benga when he relocated to Virginia, working tirelessly to restore his autonomy and human dignity.

Anne Spencer: The celebrated African American poet and civil rights activist based in Lynchburg, Virginia, who befriended and tutored Ota Benga. Spencer offered intellectual companionship and emotional support, helping Benga navigate life away from the trauma of the exhibition circuit while connecting him with broader networks of Black intellectual resistance.

African American Newspapers and Editors: Editorial boards across the United States—including prominent Black-owned publications such as the New York Age and other national journals—waged an unyielding media campaign against the exhibitions. Editors like Reverend Matthew Gilbert forcefully dismantled the racist justifications promoted by mainstream outlets like The New York Times, exposing the hypocrisy of a society that claimed to champion progress while practicing modern barbarism.

Archival Reports and Eyewitness Documentations

The documentary footprint of human exhibitions reveals how institutionalized racism was systematically operationalized, recorded, and defended through administrative reports, municipal logs, and contemporary press correspondence.

The St. Louis World's Fair Commission Reports (1904): Official administrative documents from the Louisiana Purchase Exposition detailed the precise logistical management of the 47-acre Philippine Reservation. Bureaucrats tracked indigenous participants—including Igorot, Negrito, and Bontoc groups—not as human beings, but as inventory. Reports documented daily caloric rations, housing conditions, and medical isolations, treating human endurance as quantifiable data for imperial study.

The New York Zoological Society Administrative Files: Internal correspondence between zoo directors, curators, and eugenicists like Madison Grant exposed the calculated mechanics behind Ota Benga's 1906 display in the primate house. Archives contained drafts of promotional signage, attendance logs showing over 40,000 daily visitors, and memos outlining strategies to deflect humanitarian criticism by framing the spectacle as an "anthropological lesson".

Eyewitness Press Dispatches: Newspaper accounts from the era captured the raw hostility of the environment. Reporters from major metropolitan dailies described how crowds would gawk, jeer, and throw objects at captives, while independent black-press journalists documented the deep psychological distress, resistance, and despair experienced by those forced onto the exhibition circuit.

The Historical Record and Documentation of Atrocity

The historical documentation surrounding the human exhibition era provides undeniable proof of how municipal bodies, academic societies, and federal governments coordinated the public commodification of human beings. Archival reports, exposition commissions, and institutional records preserve the mechanics of these spectacles, detailing everything from logistical transit manifests to public relations strategies designed to manufacture consensus.

The Tervuren Colonial Section Records (1897): Archival files from the International Exhibition in Brussels—established at the behest of King Leopold II—meticulously documented the forced relocation of 267 Congolese men, women, and children into artificial fenced "villages". These reports tracked daily attendance figures peaking at over 40,000 visitors a day, alongside the grim medical logs recording the deaths of individuals such as Sambo, Mpemba, Ngemba, Ekia, Nzau, Kitukwa, and Mibange, whose lives were sacrificed for Belgian colonial propaganda.

The Louisiana Purchase Exposition Archives (1904): Administrative records from the St. Louis World's Fair preserved the blueprint of the 47-acre Philippine Reservation. Bureaucrats filed exhaustive inventories detailing the housing, dietary rations, and behavioral oversight of over 1,100 indigenous Filipinos, reducing complex human populations to quantifiable data points for imperial study and exhibition management.

The Wildlife Conservation Society and Zoological Archives: Internal correspondence between New York Zoological Society leaders, administrators, and eugenicists revealed the calculated framing of Ota Benga's 1906 confinement in the Bronx Zoo primate house. Memos, promotional drafts, and visitor logs demonstrated how institutional authorities deliberately marketed human suffering as an "educational anthropology lesson" while deflecting moral outrage through the shield of academic prestige.

The Human Stories Behind the Spectacle

Beyond the cold administrative ledgers, institutional memos, and newspaper editorials lie the deeply personal, tragic narratives of individuals whose lives were upended by the machinery of human exhibitions. These personal accounts capture the profound human cost of an era defined by clinical detachment and imperial ambition.

Ota Benga's Journey and Internal Turmoil: snatched from his home in the Congo Free State by slave traders and later purchased by anthropologist Samuel Phillips Verner, Ota Benga's life became a harrowing testament to the cruelty of the era. Beyond the days spent caged in the Bronx Zoo primate house, archival accounts and personal testimonies revealed a man trapped in a profound state of displacement. Though freed from the zoo through the fierce advocacy of Black clergymen, Benga struggled intensely with his inability to return home due to the ongoing violence in the

Congo under King Leopold's regime. The psychological weight of public humiliation, coupled with the tragic realization of his permanent separation from his homeland and family, drove him to deep despair, culminating in his tragic death by suicide in Virginia in 1916.

The Resistance and Resilience of the Igorot Villagers: At the 1904 St. Louis World's Fair, the Igorot contingent from the Philippines was subjected to relentless public scrutiny, cultural degradation, and extreme weather. Despite being forced into humiliating routines—such as the sensationalized, daily public consumption of dogs to satisfy American expectations of "savagery"—the villagers maintained a quiet, steadfast dignity. Archival notes and oral histories passed down through generations reveal that the Igorot people actively resisted their commodification by refusing to perform on certain days, staging silent protests, and demanding better adherence to their contractual wages from exploitative showmen. When rogue impresarios attempted to abandon their destitute in foreign cities like Ghent following the fair's conclusion, the community banded together, relying on mutual aid and sheer resilience to survive and eventually find a path back to their ancestral homes in the Cordillera mountains.

The Forgotten Lives of the Tervuren Congolese: Among the 267 Congolese individuals brought to Belgium for the 1897 International Exposition, the personal tragedy of individuals like Zao, a young mother, and several others is preserved only through the haunting medical logs and cemetery records of Tervuren. Torn from their villages and thrust into damp, freezing European weather wearing traditional attire wholly unsuited for the climate, these individuals faced rapid illness and death. Their personal narratives were systematically erased by administrators who recorded their passing merely as statistical drop-offs in daily attendance revenues. Yet, through historical recovery projects, modern descendants and historians continue to unearth their names, restoring their humanity and ensuring they are remembered not as museum curiosities, but as sovereign human beings whose lives were tragically cut short by imperial cruelty.

The Living Echo in the Modern World

The cages of the Bronx Zoo have long since been dismantled, the Philippine Reservation at St. Louis has faded into overgrown parkland, and the artificial Congolese village of Tervuren has been replaced by modern halls of research and diplomacy. Yet, the core danger that caused these atrocities has not vanished; it has merely evolved.

When digital algorithms are trained to profile marginalized populations, when human lives are reduced to quantifiable engagement metrics on screens, and when the vulnerable are packaged for voyeuristic digital consumption, the old spirit of the exhibition hall finds new life. The legacy of Ota Benga, of the Igorot villagers, and of the countless unnamed souls displayed for the amusement of the powerful stands as an urgent, ongoing warning. It reminds humanity that whenever science, technology, or governance abandon empathy, progress dissolves into tyranny—and that the fight to defend absolute human dignity is an eternal, unbroken duty.

The Final Vow

As the archives are unsealed and the hidden names of the displaced are finally spoken aloud, history delivers its ultimate verdict on the era of human exhibitions. The spectacle of the fairgrounds and the clinical coldness of the laboratories did not merely expose the cruelty of their architects; they revealed the fragile state of any civilization that places empirical ambition above human empathy.

The ghosts of Tervuren, St. Louis, and the Bronx do not ask for pity; they demand remembrance, accountability, and an unyielding commitment to justice. Their endurance through the darkest machinery of objectification serves as a timeless compass for humanity. It is a permanent reminder that true progress can never be measured by what we conquer, catalog, or display, but only by how fiercely we protect the sacred, unalienable dignity of every human soul. The ledger of the past is closed, but the vigilance required to keep its dark history from repeating remains forever unbroken.

Part II

A Nurse Looks Inside the Cage

Chapter 5

Hunger, Climate, and Disease

The human body, when subjected to the systematic calculations of colonial exhibition administration, became an experimental theater of biological vulnerability. Chapter 5 explores the granular physical realities of those confined within human zoos, world fairs, and ethnological displays. It analyzes how structured malnutrition, environmental shock, rampantly unchecked infectious diseases, and structural sanitation failures coalesced into an apparatus of slow physical destruction.

Nutritional Subversion and the Mechanics of Starvation

The deliberate manipulation of food was one of the most effective and quiet instruments of control wielded by exposition managers. Captives were rarely provided with provisions that matched their metabolic needs or cultural biochemistry.

The Replacement of Traditional Sustenance: Indigenous groups whose traditional diets relied on specialized, nutrient-rich local proteins, fresh flora, and diverse caloric sources were abruptly shifted onto cheap, bulk-purchased carbohydrates and preserved provisions. Flour, lard, sugar, and low-grade salted meats became the foundation of daily rations.

Economic Retrenchment by Showmen: Impresarios operating traveling human exhibitions viewed food as a primary operational expense to be minimized. Archival ledgers from private traveling troupes in Europe and North America consistently demonstrate that daily food budgets for exhibited individuals were fractionally lower than those allocated for the circus animals housed in adjacent enclosures.

Metabolic Collateral: This chronic under-provisioning triggered immediate physical deterioration. Muscle waste, anemia, lethargy, and severe vitamin deficiencies quickly set in. Organizers often weaponized this resulting weakness, pointing to the emaciated or exhausted states of the captives as "empirical proof" of their supposed biological inferiority, completing a circular logic of abuse.

Environmental Incompatibility and Thermal Trauma

The forced displacement of human beings across distinct climatic zones without adequate shelter or seasonal protection caused catastrophic rates of thermal shock.

Tropical Bodies in Northern Latitudes: Populations indigenous to equatorial or tropical regions—such as the Congo basin, sub-Saharan Africa, and the lowland Philippines—were routinely transported to northern European or North American exhibition grounds. They arrived equipped only with traditional light clothing suited for year-round warmth.

The Architecture of Exposure: Exhibition architecture prioritized theatrical staging over human survival. Captives were housed in open-air mock villages, drafty wooden shacks, or uninsulated canvas tents designed to mimic native conditions for the audience's aesthetic pleasure. During sudden autumnal cold snaps, heavy rainstorms, or harsh winter freezes, these structures offered zero thermal protection.

Physiological Collapse: The human body responds to abrupt, sustained cold stress through severe vasoconstriction, increased metabolic demand, and immune suppression. Without warm garments, heavy bedding, or adequate heating fuels, exhibited individuals suffered continuous cycles of hypothermia, frostbite, and rapid pulmonary distress.

Pathogenic Vulnerability and Epidemic Vectors

Exhibition sites operated as dense, unnatural epidemiological incubators where naïve populations encountered heavily mutated urban pathogen pools.

Immunological Naivety: Isolated indigenous communities possessed no ancestral or acquired immunity against the dense viral and bacterial loads circulating through Western urban centers. Pathogens that caused mild or manageable illness in European populations proved aggressively lethal to the captives.

Tuberculosis as an Executioner: Archival medical records and municipal death registers identify tuberculosis as the single most devastating killer within human exhibitions. The combination of damp, unventilated quarters, physical exhaustion from endless daily performances, and chronic malnutrition provided an ideal environment for Mycobacterium tuberculosis to spread unchecked through entire groups.

Secondary Infections and Complications: Measles, influenza, smallpox, and pneumonia swept through exhibition encampments with terrifying speed. Because public ticket sales depended on a full cast of performers, sick individuals were frequently forced to continue appearing before crowds while running high fevers, drastically accelerating their physical decline.

Sanitation Breakdown and Waterborne Pathology

Infrastructure within temporary world fairs and permanent zoological parks routinely ignored basic sanitary standards for human habitation.

The Absence of Waste Management: Encampments housing hundreds of individuals lacked functional sewage systems, greywater drainage, or safe latrine protocols. Human waste accumulated near living quarters, contaminating shallow soil beds and localized air currents.

Contaminated Water Supplies: Drinking water was frequently drawn from compromised local sources or stagnant ponds within exposition grounds. This led directly to explosive, recurrent outbreaks of waterborne diseases, including cholera, dysentery, and severe typhoid infections.

Medical Concealment and Quarantine: When epidemics broke out among the displayed groups, exposition directors and municipal health boards frequently prioritized public relations over patient care. Sick individuals were covertly transferred to hidden field hospitals or isolated off-site shacks to prevent panic among paying visitors and protect gate receipts. When patients died, their bodies were quietly processed through coroner offices with falsified cause-of-death entries designed to obscure the unsanitary conditions of the exhibition grounds.

Post-Mortem and Archival Proof of Neglect

The ultimate documentation of the physical devastation wrought by human exhibitions is found in the clinical registers, autopsy reports, and post-mortem examinations conducted by contemporary physicians. Far from being shielded by the medical ethics of their time, exhibited individuals were routinely viewed by institutional doctors as biological novelties even in death.

Autopsy Protocols and Anatomical Collection: When captives succumbed to the combined effects of malnutrition, cold exposure, and infectious disease, their bodies were frequently intercepted by university medical departments, eugenic research societies, and anthropological museums. Rather than returning remains to grieving families or native communities, institutional anatomists performed unauthorized post-mortems to measure cranial capacity, dissect organs, and preserve skeletal remains for permanent racial classification displays.

The Falsification of Medical Records: Municipal health inspectors and exposition doctors often collaborated to obfuscate the true causes of death on official certificates. Terms like "general debility," "natural causes," or vague tropical fevers were systematically substituted for starvation, severe hypothermia, advanced tuberculosis, and cholera. This administrative deception protected organizers from civil liability, criminal prosecution, and public outrage.

The Legacy of Biological Exploitation: The medical files and autopsy logs preserved in state archives serve as an unyielding indictment of an era where scientific curiosity completely eclipsed basic human empathy. They stand as permanent testimony to how systematic physical neglect was officially coded as routine administrative management, leaving a dark blueprint of institutional indifference that modern medicine and anthropology continue to confront today.

The Clinical Gaze and Anthropometric Examination

The physical examination of individuals trapped within human exhibitions was never an act of genuine healthcare. Instead, it was an intrusive, clinical ritual designed to feed the pseudoscience of racial typologies, craniometry, and evolutionary ranking. Whenever doctors, anthropologists, or exposition officials turned their attention to the health of the captives, their methods transformed human bodies into experimental objects.

Anthropometric Measurements as Health Checks: Routine physical checkups were co-opted by eugenicists and physical anthropologists who cared little for the wellness of the captives. Instead of treating symptoms of exhaustion or malnutrition, examiners used calipers, tape measures, and scale weights to record cranial dimensions, limb lengths, facial angles, and body fat distribution. These invasive measurements were cataloged alongside disease logs to establish a supposed hierarchy of human evolution.

Invasive Public Examinations: Exhibited individuals were frequently subjected to public medical demonstrations. Spectators paying admission to world fairs or ethnographic shows could watch doctors inspect captives' teeth, skin, and muscles on elevated stages, treating physical bodies as exotic biological exhibits. Medical students and professors were often given exclusive access behind the scenes to conduct humiliating physical surveys without consent.

Post-Mortem Medical Salvage: When illness, exposure, or starvation proved fatal, the clinical examination escalated to its most macabre phase. Rather than providing compassionate end-of-life care or respectful burials, institutional physicians treated dying and deceased captives as immediate research opportunities. Autopsies were rushed not to determine cures, but to harvest brains, bones, and soft tissue samples for permanent display in European and American university anatomical collections.

The Pathological Catalog of the Exhibition Circuit

The closed environment of human exhibitions created a breeding ground for specific, devastating pathogens. Historical medical registries, municipal health board filings, and contemporary physician logs document a horrifying spectrum of diseases that swept through the encampments, systematically exploiting the weakened immune systems, malnutrition, and thermal shock of the captives.

Primary Pathological Killers

Medical documentation from world fairs, colonial expositions, and zoological displays consistently highlights several specific infectious diseases as the primary causes of morbidity and mortality among exhibited groups:

Tuberculosis (Mycobacterium tuberculosis): By far the most lethal disease within exhibition grounds. Driven by unventilated, damp living quarters (such as the makeshift huts at the Tervuren colonial exhibition or the poorly insulated quarters at the St. Louis World's Fair), exhaustion from daily performances, and chronic malnutrition, tuberculosis tore through groups with relentless speed. It is frequently manifested in both pulmonary forms and extrapulmonary systemic infections.

Pneumonia and Acute Respiratory Infections: Because tropical and equatorial populations were thrust into freezing European and North American climates without adequate clothing or heating, upper respiratory infections rapidly escalated into fatal pneumonias. The sudden drop in temperature paralyzed mucociliary clearance in the lungs, allowing bacterial pneumonia to take hold within days.

Cholera and Waterborne Dysentery: The catastrophic failure of sanitation infrastructure on exhibition sites—marked by unmanaged waste and contaminated drinking water—triggered explosive outbreaks of Asiatic cholera and bacillary dysentery. These waterborne illnesses caused severe dehydration, electrolyte collapse, and rapid death within hours of symptom onset.

Measles and Varicella (Chickenpox): Due to strict historical isolation from urban European pathogen pools, many indigenous groups possessed complete immunological naivety to common childhood diseases. When introduced into the crowded exhibition camps, measles acted as a hyper-virulent killer, causing severe systemic inflammation, secondary pneumonia, and high mortality rates.

Smallpox: Though occasionally mitigated by forced or quarantine measures, smallpox outbreaks remained a constant, terrifying threat in densely populated exposition zones where thousands of external visitors mingled daily with the captive performers.

Malaria and Tropical Fevers: Many individuals arrived carrying chronic, latent protozoan infections from their native regions. Stripped of adequate nutrition, exhausted by grueling schedules, and suffering from systemic stress, these latent infections flared up violently, compounded by secondary opportunistic pathogens.

The Clinical Exploitation of Sickness

When these diseases inevitably struck, the medical personnel assigned to the exhibitions rarely acted as healers. Instead, medical officers documented the progression of these exact pathologies as "proof" of racial vulnerability or natural selection. Autopsy registers from institutions tied to world's fairs reveal that physicians closely studied how tuberculosis and dysentery ravaged non-Western bodies, treating the agonizing symptoms of structural neglect as biological data points for the expansion of scientific racism.

The Shadow of Medical Experimentation and Pharmacological Trials

Beyond observing the natural progression of epidemics, institutional physicians and university-backed researchers occasionally crossed the line from passive documentation into active medical experimentation. Shielded by the legal impunity of exposition management and the total dehumanization of the captives, clinical sites on exhibition grounds occasionally functioned as testing grounds for unproven treatments, vaccines, and pharmaceutical interventions.

Experimental Vaccinations and Serums: Historical records from late 19th- and early 20th-century colonial exhibitions indicate that when outbreaks of smallpox, cholera, or typhoid threatened public attendance and ticket sales, medical officers sometimes administered experimental, unrefined vaccines or antitoxins directly to captive populations without informed consent. Because these biological agents were frequently untested on immunologically naive groups, they often provoked severe adverse reactions, systemic toxicity, and accelerated organ failure rather than protection.

Nutritional Deficiency Trials: As captive populations succumbed to widespread scurvy, beriberi, and severe protein-energy malnutrition due to substandard rations, institutional doctors occasionally used these controlled environments to observe the physiological limits of starvation. Rather than correcting the dietary intake, researchers cataloged the exact timeline of muscle atrophy, cognitive decline, and metabolic collapse, treating human suffering as a fixed clinical variable.

The Suppression of Whistleblower Accounts: Occasionally, independent physicians, visiting nurses, or foreign human rights observers voiced alarm over the rampant disease and neglect inside the encampments. Exhibition directors, fearing financial ruin and political scandal, systematically discredited these accounts, barring independent inspections and threatening whistleblowers with legal retaliation or revocation of their exhibition credentials. The medical narrative was strictly managed to protect the economic engine of the spectacle, ensuring that the true cost of hunger, climate shock, and disease remained buried beneath layers of bureaucratic cover-ups and pseudoscientific rationalization.

Inside the Isolation Tents and Sick Wards of the Fairgrounds

When illness inevitably struck the encampments of the world's fairs and colonial expositions, the administrative machinery shifted from public spectacle to hidden containment. The reality of a sick performer threatening the illusion of "primitive wonder" meant that illness was handled not through compassionate healthcare, but through concealment, institutional callousness, and forced isolation.

The Anatomy of the Fairground Sick Tent

Behind the simulated native villages, thatched huts, and fenced compounds lay makeshift medical facilities—often referred to as field hospitals, isolation shacks, or quarantine tents.

Concealment from the Public Eye: Fair organizers meticulously protected the paying public from the grim realities of human suffering. If a performer contracted tuberculosis, pneumonia, or cholera, they were quickly removed from the main exhibition loop. Ill individuals were transferred to damp, unheated back-stage tents or off-site municipal wards where visitors could not witness the physical toll of the exposition.

The Continuation of Forced Labor Under Duress: Because troupes were under strict contractual obligations—and showmen wanted to avoid the expense of idle performers or emergency replacements—sick individuals were frequently forced to continue performing while experiencing high fevers, racking coughs, and severe physical weakness. Archival notes from European and American fairs describe performers wrapped in hidden blankets or given stimulants just long enough to endure a daily public demonstration before collapsing back into their quarters.

The Role of Fairground Doctors: Physicians stationed at these exhibitions were primarily contracted by management to protect public health optics, not the welfare of the captives. Their daily logs focus heavily on containing contagion to prevent municipal shutdowns and maintaining a minimum threshold of able-bodied performers to keep the box office operational.

Specific Historical Instances of Fairground Illness and Isolation

The St. Louis World's Fair Epidemic Shocks (1904): Within the 47-acre Philippine Reservation, the transition from tropical climates to the volatile Missouri weather—marked by severe summer heatwaves followed by sudden, chilling rains—wreaked havoc on the inhabitants. Archival records from the exhibition's hospital tent document numerous cases of severe respiratory infections, dysentery, and measles among the Bontoc, Igorot, and Visayan participants. When individuals fell critically ill, they were isolated in makeshift medical tents where limited supplies and cold floors accelerated their decline. Several participants who succumbed to these illnesses were buried in temporary graves far from home before their families even received clear word of their conditions.

The Tervuren Cholera and Influenza Scares (1897): At the Brussels International Exposition in Belgium, the makeshift Congolese village became a focal point of public health panic when damp weather and contaminated water sources triggered widespread dysentery and severe influenza. Rather than evacuating the participants to proper European medical facilities, Belgian authorities established a strict quarantine around the village, barring outside journalists and human rights observers. Medical logs from the site reveal that sick individuals were treated with basic, ineffective palliatives while the exhibition continued to admit thousands of daily visitors unaware of the biological crisis unfolding behind the fences.

The Traveling Ethnological Troupes: In private, commercial human zoos that toured European capitals, illness was treated as a financial liability. When members of traveling African or Indigenous troupes fell ill with tuberculosis or smallpox, they were frequently abandoned in foreign municipal hospitals by bankrupt or fleeing impresarios. Left in unfamiliar cities without translators, money, or advocacy, these abandoned performers faced institutional neglect, with their final days documented only in cold municipal coroner reports thousands of miles from their birthplaces.

The Anatomy of the Examiners

When illness breached the encampments, who examined the captives? The medical gatekeepers of the human exhibitions were not independent healers; they were institutional agents whose professional loyalties lay with exposition management, academic societies, and the state. A distinct hierarchy of examiners dictated the fate of the sick:

Exposition-Contracted Physicians: These doctors were hired directly by fair syndicates or private showmen. Their primary mandate was operational protection: determining whether a sick performer was contagious enough to warrant quarantine or functional enough to be pushed back onto the exhibition stage. They functioned as risk managers rather than clinicians.

University Anthropologists and Physical Scientists: Researchers from academic institutions frequently bypassed bedside care altogether to conduct anthropometric surveys on ailing subjects. They viewed the hospital tents and quarantine wards as rare laboratories where they could chart the final stages of racial theories, measuring pulse rates, fever progression, and wasting muscles as scientific data points.

State and Municipal Health Officers: Local government inspectors entered the encampments only when an outbreak threatened to spill over into the surrounding civilian population. Their interventions were designed to protect the tax-paying citizenry through forced quarantine or rapid concealment, completely ignoring the underlying structural causes of the illness.

Deprived of compassionate advocates, the sick captives faced an apparatus where examination was merely a prelude to either forced labor or clinical post-mortem salvage.

Archival records detailing the medical conditions, treatment, and mortality of specific groups kept in human exhibitions do exist, though they were typically maintained as administrative logs, municipal health files, or anthropological data sets rather than patient-centric health records.

The 1904 St. Louis World's Fair Files: Records preserved in state historical archives and municipal libraries include official hospital registers, camp infirmary logs, and vaccination records detailing the treatment—and frequent lack thereof—administered to indigenous performers within the Philippine Reservation and other ethnological displays. These documents outline outbreaks of measles, dysentery, and respiratory infections, alongside the names of individuals who passed away in field hospitals.

University and Museum Anthropometric Collections: Institutions such as the Field Museum and various university departments house extensive physical and biological data—including anthropometric measurements, dental casts, and hair or tissue samples—collected from indigenous groups during major expositions like the 1893 Chicago World's Columbian Exposition.

Colonial Exposition Death Registers: Archival registries from events like the 1897 Brussels International Exposition in Tervuren contain specific mortality logs and cemetery records documenting the tragic passing of Congolese participants, which administrators initially attempted to obscure beneath sanitized public relations reports.

Recovering the Named Dead from the Archives

The grim reality of these medical failures and institutional records is anchored by specific, recovered names that cut through the anonymous statistics of the exhibition circuit. Historical recovery projects across Europe and North America have successfully brought to light precise documentation of those who perished under the weight of climate shock, disease, and neglect.

The Tervuren Registry (1897): Historical documentation preserved regarding King Leopold II's colonial exhibition in Tervuren, Belgium, records the tragic fates of individuals such as Ekia, Gemba, Kitukwa, Mpela, Zao, Samba, and Mbange. These seven Congolese individuals—among the 267 transported to the exhibition—succumbed to severe pneumonia, influenza, and acute respiratory distress brought on by freezing, damp Belgian weather and inadequate housing. Their deaths, initially obscured in administrative ledgers as minor demographic fluctuations, are now permanently marked next to the parish church of Sint-Jan Evangelist in Tervuren, restoring identity to the victims of pathological neglect.

The Antwerp World Fair Records (1894): Archival discoveries concerning the 1894 Antwerp exposition detail the deaths of participants such as Sabo, Bitio, Isokoyé, Manguesse, Binda, Mangwanda, and Pezo, who perished shortly after arrival due to a combination of exposure, viral infections, and systemic exhaustion. Medical and municipal tracking showed that upon death, their remains were treated with institutional callousness, eventually relegated to unmarked collective spaces until modern historical investigations brought their fates back into public awareness.

The St. Louis Philippine Reservation Logs (1904): Official historical documentation and camp hospital logs from the 47-acre Philippine Reservation at the St. Louis World's Fair record approximately 17 deaths among the indigenous participants. Caused primarily by advanced pneumonia, severe malnutrition, and a complete lack of immunity to local pathogen pools, these fatalities were meticulously recorded by camp physicians and administrators who nonetheless continued to prioritize public ticket sales and structural operations over emergency medical evacuation or culturally responsive care.

The Pharmacies of Neglect and Unproven Cures

When illness overwhelmed the camps, the medical treatments available to the captives were defined by the limitations of late 19th- and early 20th-science, compounded by institutional cruelty. The medicines administered in the fairground sick tents were rarely designed to cure; instead, they were blunt instruments meant to suppress symptoms, enforce compliance, or test chemical agents.

Alkaloids, Opiates, and Heavy Sedatives: Standard medical arsenals of the era relied heavily on patent medicines, alcohol-based tinctures, and powerful narcotics like liquid laudanum and morphine. When performers suffered from agonizing symptoms of tuberculosis, severe coughing fits, or freezing chills, camp physicians frequently administered heavy sedatives or opiates. These drugs did not treat the underlying infections; they merely numbed the patients, rendering sick individuals compliant and quiet while keeping them operational for the daily exhibition schedule.

Primitive Antipyretics and Harsh Palliatives: Quinine was widely dispensed for tropical fevers or suspected malaria flare-ups, though often in unregulated or incorrect dosages that caused severe side effects, including hearing loss, gastrointestinal distress, and dizziness. For respiratory distress and lung inflammation, doctors used counterirritants like mustard plasters, blistering agents, or crude expectorants that caused intense physical pain without curing the underlying pneumonia.

The Withholding of Advanced Therapeutics: While breakthrough treatments and antiseptic protocols were beginning to emerge in elite Western hospitals during this era, they were rarely deployed in exhibition infirmaries. Captives were denied access to proper convalescent care, nourishing diets, or clean environments. Medicine inside the human zoos was treated as a rationed commodity—distributed sparingly, weaponized for control, and ultimately powerless against the systemic devastation of climate shock, starvation, and infectious disease.

Traditional Natural Remedies Versus Western Clinical Palliatives

When the medical apparatus of the human exhibitions failed the captives, individuals trapped within the camps frequently attempted to rely on their own ancestral knowledge, traditional pharmacopeia, and natural healing methods. However, this collision between indigenous healing practices and Western exhibition management created a tense, restrictive dynamic within the camp confines.

The Suppression and Appropriation of Traditional Remedies

Indigenous performers arriving from Africa, Asia, and the Americas often brought traditional herbal medicines, botanical preparations, and holistic healing protocols suited for their native environments. These natural remedies were systematically disrupted or forbidden by camp authorities:

Confiscation of Botanical Supplies: Exhibition inspectors and camp security frequently searched for the personal belongings of incoming groups, confiscating dried herbs, roots, barks, and traditional healing implements under the guise of maintaining camp hygiene or preventing the introduction of "unauthorized" substances. Showmen feared that traditional rituals or remedies might frighten paying visitors or disrupt the fabricated illusion of raw, uncultivated savagery.

Denial of Access to Natural Ingredients: Even when performers attempted to forage or replicate traditional remedies locally, the foreign urban ecosystems of northern European and American fairgrounds offered none of the specific flora, fauna, or mineral components required for their traditional pharmacopeia.

Western Clinical Palliatives vs. Holistic Needs

To combat the wave of respiratory illnesses, gastrointestinal infections, and chronic pain, camp physicians relied exclusively on late 19th- and early 20th-century Western pharmacy, which often worsened the physical suffering of the captives:

Crude Mercury and Arsenic Compounds: Standard therapeutic regimens of the era frequently included toxic heavy metals. Calomel (mercurous chloride) was widely dispensed as a purgative for dysentery and stomach ailments, frequently resulting in severe mercury poisoning, mucosal tissue destruction, and agonizing dental and gastrointestinal complications.

Alcohol-Laden Tonics: Patent medicines and "cure-alls" prescribed by fairground doctors were heavily laced with high-proof alcohol, opium, or cocaine. While these substances temporarily numbed the severe physical pain of frostbite, tuberculosis, and exhaustion, they rapidly compromised the patients' already failing immune systems and induced chemical dependency.

Ineffective Counterirritants: For severe chest congestion and early-stage pneumonia caused by freezing exhibition huts, doctors applied blistering plasters made from mustard seed or Spanish fly (Cantharis). These remedies caused painful chemical burns on the skin in a futile effort to draw inflammation away from the lungs, providing zero therapeutic benefit while adding physical trauma to an already dying patient.

The Ultimate Breakdown of Bodily Resilience

As the weeks of the exhibitions stretched on, the cumulative weight of nutritional deprivation, thermal shock, untreated infectious diseases, and toxic Western palliatives brought the captives to the absolute limits of human endurance. The final days of those who fell ill were marked by a profound institutional abandonment that exposed the darkest core of the exhibition enterprise.

The Final Stages of Wasting: Autopsy logs and clinical notes from exhibition infirmaries document rapid, catastrophic body weight loss among chronic tuberculosis and dysentery patients. Stripped of traditional protective fats and proteins, and given only low-grade, bulk-purchased carbohydrates, patients suffered from advanced cachexia—muscle atrophy so severe that contemporary physicians recorded it in clinical journals as an anatomical curiosity rather than a medical emergency.

The Silence of the Final Hours: When death finally arrived in the quarantine tents or makeshift back-stage shacks, it occurred in profound isolation. Denied access to their spiritual leaders, traditional mourning rites, or family members—who were often forced to continue performing for paying crowds just outside the medical tent—the dying spent their final moments surrounded by institutional machinery that viewed their passing as little more than a logistical inconvenience.

The Erasure of Identity in Death: Even after death, the physical bodies of the captives were denied peace. Instead of receiving dignified burials within their cultural traditions, many corpses were transferred directly to medical colleges, anthropological research societies, and museum vaults. There, their bones, brains, and tissue samples were cataloged and placed on permanent display, completing a cycle where human beings were exploited in life, neglected in illness, and commodified even after death.

Additional Historical Milestones of Pathological Neglect

To fully understand the systemic scope of how disease and environmental shock weaponized human exhibitions, several other well-documented historical instances reveal the identical patterns of institutional neglect, medical exploitation, and administrative cover-ups across global exposition sites.

The 1906 Bronx Zoo Ota Benga Crisis

The notorious display of Ota Benga, an Mbuti Congolese man, at the New York Zoological Park (Bronx Zoo) in 1906 highlights how physical and psychological stress intersected under the guise of public science:

The Pathological Intersection of Captivity and Trauma: While Benga was not documented as suffering from a major epidemic disease during his initial weeks in the zoo's monkey house, the severe psychological trauma of captivity compounded by physical exhaustion led to profound behavioral and physiological decline.

Medical and Institutional Complicity: Zoological directors, led by William Hornaday, collaborated with prominent eugenicists like Madison Grant to frame Benga's physical stature and dental modifications as evolutionary anomalies. When religious leaders and public welfare advocates finally protested the inhumane exhibition, zoo administrators and city health officials scrambled to medically clear Benga, treating public outrage as a public relations hurdle rather than an ethical violation.

Subsequent Health Decline: Following his removal from public display, Benga was shifted through various institutional settings, including the Howard Colored Orphan Asylum. Displaced from his homeland, unable to return to the Congo due to wartime travel restrictions, and suffering from severe, untreated depression and profound alienation, Benga ultimately took his own life in 1916—a delayed casualty of exhibition exploitation.

The 1931 Paris Colonial Exposition (Exposition Coloniale Internationale)

Decades after the Tervuren and St. Louis exhibitions, the 1931 Paris Colonial Exposition proved that the medical maltreatment of exhibited humans had not evolved, despite modern medical advancements:

Massive Scale and Pathogenic Density: Housing thousands of indigenous participants from French colonies across Africa, Asia, and the Pacific, the sprawling Bois de Vincennes site functioned as an immense biological theater. Participants were housed in hastily constructed "authentic" villages that lacked modern sanitation, forcing them to rely on contaminated local water sources.

Typhoid and Respiratory Outbreaks: Archival health files from the Paris exhibition document significant outbreaks of typhoid fever, severe influenza, and acute pulmonary infections among West African and Indochinese participants.

The Suppression of Morbidity Data: Fearing that news of widespread illness would disrupt the exposition's political mission to showcase the "success" of the French colonial empire, organizers utilized military quarantine protocols. Sick performers were swiftly moved to hidden military field hospitals on the periphery of Paris. Deaths were systematically downplayed in official government reports, ensuring that the human cost of imperial pageantry remained hidden behind state propaganda.

The Pan-American Exposition in Buffalo (1901)

The 1901 exposition in Buffalo, New York, featured extensive "Indian Congress" and ethnological displays where indigenous groups from the American West and various global territories were assembled under harsh climatic conditions:

Environmental and Dietary Disruption: Participants were subjected to erratic weather shifts typical of Western New York, moving from oppressive summer heatwaves to sudden, damp lake-effect chills. The processed rations provided by exposition contractors failed to meet the metabolic needs of the performers, triggering widespread gastrointestinal distress and severe fatigue.

Measles and Scarlet Fever Spreads: Historical health records from the exposition's medical tent note concentrated outbreaks of childhood infectious diseases, exacerbated by the dense mingling of visitors and the lack of proper ventilation in the encampments. When individuals fell severely ill, they faced rapid isolation, minimal clinical intervention, and quiet administrative processing if the illness proved fatal.

Further Historical Documentation of Exhibition Pathology

The historical archive is replete with additional case studies that reinforce the systemic patterns of nutritional deprivation, climate shock, and medical exploitation across the global human exhibition circuit.

The 1889 Paris Universal Exposition (Exposition Universelle)

The monumental 1889 exposition in Paris, which famously featured the Village Nègre housing 400 indigenous individuals, established a dark blueprint for subsequent world's fairs regarding health management:

Inadequate Shelter and Thermal Stress: Participants from tropical and sub-Saharan regions were housed in temporary enclosures that provided minimal defense against the damp, unpredictable Parisian autumn weather. Archival records from the exhibition's auxiliary medical posts note rapid occurrences of severe chest colds, bronchitis, and early-stage pulmonary infections within weeks of the opening.

Exploitation of the Sick for Spectacle: Because the Village Nègre was one of the most financially lucrative attractions of the 1889 fair, organizers placed immense pressure on participants to maintain daily schedules. Even individuals running high fevers or suffering from debilitating gastrointestinal distress were coerced into performing traditional dances and crafts under the threat of financial penalties or withholding of meager daily rations.

The 1924 British Empire Exhibition at Wembley

Decades into the 20th century, major imperial showcases continued to treat human participants as expendable biological assets rather than human beings requiring medical protection:

Nutritional Neglect and Dietary Collapse: Participants brought from various African and Asian territories to populate the exhibition's imperial villages were subjected to rigid, low-cost catering contracts managed by exposition accountants. The resulting dietary monotony triggered widespread vitamin deficiencies, dramatic weight loss, and general lethargy among the troupes.

Covert Medical Repatriation: When illness became severe—particularly cases of advanced tuberculosis or chronic respiratory failure—exposition authorities routinely avoided local public health scrutiny by hastily arranging emergency transport or paying for quiet repatriations. The goal was to ensure that deaths occurred outside the host country's municipal jurisdiction, thereby manipulating public mortality statistics and maintaining the illusion of a pristine imperial spectacle.

The Institutional Architecture of Silence and Complicity

To fully comprehend the medical catastrophe of the human exhibition era, one must examine the institutional architecture that allowed widespread suffering, disease, and death to persist in plain sight. The collaboration between municipal authorities, academic institutions, exposition syndicates, and corporate sponsors created a fortress of bureaucratic indifference.

The Bureaucracy of Concealment

When human beings were imported into European and American exhibition grounds, their legal status was deliberately left ambiguous. They were neither recognized as fully autonomous citizens with labor rights nor treated as traditional hospital patients with protected medical privacy. This legal vacuum enabled organizers to construct a comprehensive system of administrative concealment:

Internal Censorship of Camp Journals: Daily operational logs maintained by exposition managers frequently omitted references to illness, worker strikes, or declining health. When internal memorandums mentioned outbreaks of disease, they were coded in clinical, detached language that prioritized financial risk assessment over human welfare. Words like "attrition," "unfitness," and "replacement units" were routinely substituted for diagnoses of tuberculosis, starvation, and hypothermia.

Collaboration with Local Press: Exhibition press offices maintained tight control over journalists and photographers allowed inside the camp perimeters. Reporters were guided along curated pathways, strictly barred from entering isolation tents or field infirmaries. Any journalist who attempted to independently investigate camp mortality rates or interview sick performers faced immediate credential revocation and public defamation by syndicate PR campaigns.

The Manipulation of Death Certificates: To bypass municipal health codes and avoid negative publicity, organizers often worked in tandem with sympathetic local coroners. Causes of death were systematically falsified on municipal registers. An individual who died of advanced tuberculosis induced by damp housing and malnutrition was formally recorded as dying from "natural congenital weakness" or "acclimatization failure," shifting the blame from institutional neglect to inherent biological deficiency.

The Economic Calculus of Human Exposure

At the heart of the exhibition enterprise lay a brutal economic calculation. Human zoos, colonial displays, and ethnological villages were multi-million-dollar commercial ventures driven by ticket sales, merchandise concessions, and government subsidies. In this context, human health was treated purely as an asset depreciation schedule:

The Cost-Benefit Analysis of Rations: Catering contracts for the encampments were routinely awarded to the lowest commercial bidders. Exhibition accountants calculated the absolute minimum daily caloric intake required to keep a human body upright and functional for public display. When rising food costs or supply chain disruptions squeezed profit margins, the quality and quantity of rations were immediately reduced, plunging vulnerable populations into acute malnutrition long before overt disease symptoms appeared.

The Financial Penalty of Idleness: Performers were bound by restrictive contracts that penalized them for missing performances. Illness was treated by management not as a medical emergency, but as a breach of contract. Captives forced onto the stage while running high fevers or suffering from severe physical exhaustion experienced accelerated physiological collapse, transforming a temporary, treatable infection into a terminal condition.

Insurance and Liability Evasion: Exhibition syndicates carried extensive liability policies for property damage, structural failures, and visitor accidents, but systematically excluded human performers from formal medical insurance coverage. When a participant died, contracts often contained clauses that transferred the financial burden of burial or repatriation away from the organizers, leaving destitute troupes to rely on charity or municipal pauper graves.

The Complicity of the Scientific Community

While commercial showmen profited from the ticket sales, the scientific community—specifically university departments, anthropological societies, and medical schools—provided the ideological justification and the ultimate anatomical harvest for the exhibition circuit:

Pre-Mortem Scientific Exploitation:

Academic researchers viewed the encampments as open-air laboratories. Anthropologists frequented the camps not to offer medical relief, but to recruit subjects for physiological testing.

Captives were subjected to exhausting physical evaluations, sensory threshold tests, and metabolic tracking while already weakened by poor nutrition and environmental shock. This constant intrusion drained their remaining energy reserves, accelerating their decline.

Post-Mortem Institutional Salvage: The relationship between exposition infirmaries and university anatomy departments was characterized by a seamless pipeline of biological acquisition. The moment a captive was pronounced dead, their body became the property of institutional science. Skulls were boiled and bleached, brains were preserved in formaldehyde, and complete skeletal sets were cataloged for racial comparison studies. This systematic looting of human remains ensured that the physical exploitation of the victims extended decades, and in some cases centuries, past their death.

The Long Shadow of Modern Institutions

The medical and administrative practices documented within the archives of 19th- and early 20th-century human exhibitions left a profound, unacknowledged legacy on modern scientific and medical institutions.

The Origins of Institutional Detachment: The normalization of treating marginalized populations as biological data points rather than human patients established dangerous precedents that echoed throughout 20th-century clinical trials, institutional human research, and colonial medicine. The bureaucratic distance maintained by exposition doctors—where human suffering was rationalized as scientific progress—foreshadowed later ethical breaches in medical research.

The Continuing Struggle for Repatriation: Today, indigenous communities, human rights advocates, and descendant families continue the arduous process of locating and repatriating the remains and medical artifacts harvested during the exhibition era. Museums and university archives across Europe and North America hold thousands of remains stolen from exhibition camps and field hospitals, serving as a silent, unyielding reminder of a time when hunger, climate, and disease were weaponized for public entertainment and pseudoscientific profit.

The Psychological Pathology of Exhibition Confinement

Beyond the physical ravages of tuberculosis, pneumonia, dysentery, and toxic medical palliatives, the health of individuals trapped within human exhibitions was profoundly undermined by acute psychological trauma. The intersection of forced confinement, public humiliation, cultural displacement, and constant surveillance generated a distinct psychosomatic toll that camp physicians routinely misdiagnosed or weaponized to fit racial theories.

Psychosomatic Collapse and "Nostalgia"

Late 19th- and early 20th-century medical logs frequently document profound behavioral shifts among captive performers, which European and American clinicians attempted to categorize through flawed medical frameworks:

The Pathologizing of Homesickness: Medical officers often recorded cases of severe depression, withdrawal, and refusal to eat under the outdated diagnostic term "nostalgia" or mal du pays. Rather than recognizing this as a normal human response to kidnapping, forced labor, extreme isolation, and cultural dislocation, camp doctors treated it as a congenital weakness or a psychological defect unique to non-Western peoples.

Catatonic Withdrawal and Behavioral Shutdown: Confronted daily by screaming crowds, invasive photography, and the complete stripping of personal dignity, many captives experienced severe psychological shock. Historical descriptions from camp infirmaries note individuals who stopped speaking, refused all interactions, and lapsed into catatonic states. Instead of providing psychological support or compassionate release, exposition management viewed these individuals as ruined commercial assets and relegated them to dark back-stage quarters.

The Weaponization of Mental Decline: University anthropologists and eugenicists frequently capitalized on the psychological distress of the captives. They interpreted depression, anxiety, and cognitive decline resulting from starvation and trauma as empirical "evidence" of intellectual and emotional inferiority, seamlessly feeding psychological pathology back into the pseudoscientific machinery of racial ranking.

The Total Collapse of Communal Coping Mechanisms

In their native environments, indigenous communities relied heavily on complex social structures, spiritual leadership, traditional ceremonies, and communal caregiving to process illness, grief, and physical hardship. Human exhibitions systematically destroyed these vital coping systems:

The Prohibition of Mourning and Ritual: When participants fell ill or died, camp rules strictly forbade traditional death rites, spiritual gatherings, or communal mourning. Showmen feared that authentic expressions of grief would upset paying visitors or disrupt the festive, exotic illusion of the fair. Consequently, the living was forced to suppress their sorrow and continue performing dances and daily routines while processing the loss of family members and peers.

Forced Integration of Strangers: Exhibition organizers frequently threw together disparate individuals from entirely different linguistic, cultural, and geographic backgrounds, sometimes hailing from rival or warring groups—into the same cramped compounds. This engineered friction eroded traditional social safety nets, intensified interpersonal stress, and eliminated any sense of psychological security or solidarity among the captives.

The Legacy of Unresolved Trauma

The psychological devastation endured by the survivors who managed to return home was lifelong and largely undocumented. Many returned to their native communities carrying not only chronic physical disabilities, permanent organ damage from untreated infections, and scars from unconsented medical procedures, but also deep, invisible wounds of profound betrayal. The silence enforced by exposition contracts, the loss of peers buried in foreign soil, and the enduring stigma of having been publicly displayed created generational trauma that ripple through descendant communities to this day, underscoring that the true pathology of human exhibitions was as mental as it was physical.

The Post-Mortem Economy and the Final Ledger of Exploitation

The tragic trajectory of human exhibitions did not conclude with the final breath drawn in a damp quarantine tent or a municipal isolation ward. For many of the individuals who perished under the weight of climate shock, starvation, and untreated disease, death marked the transition into a final, institutionalized phase of commodification: the post-mortem economy of human remains

The Anatomy of Post-Mortem Trafficking

When an exhibited performer succumbed to tuberculosis, pneumonia, or acute malnutrition, camp administrators and collaborating academic institutions operated with ruthless efficiency to strip the body of any remaining scientific or financial value:

The Expedited Autopsy Pipeline: University medical departments and anthropological societies maintained standing agreements with exposition syndicates. Upon a participant's death, bodies were frequently diverted away from grieving peers or religious rites directly to local medical colleges or anatomical institutes. Under the guise of establishing an official cause of death, physicians performed extensive autopsies that served a dual purpose: gathering clinical data on how non-Western bodies processed infectious diseases and harvesting skeletal or soft-tissue specimens.

The Commercialization of Skeletons and Skulls: Skeletal remains harvested from exposition casualties were meticulously cleaned, cataloged, and integrated into university osteological collections or museum exhibits across Europe and North America. Skulls were measured, drilled, and indexed to fuel the booming late 19th-century fields of craniometry and phrenology, turning the physical remnants of the deceased into permanent props for pseudoscientific racism.

The Loss of Archival Truth: To protect the reputation of the fairs and shield organizers from legal liability for criminal negligence, autopsy reports and institutional death registries were frequently falsified. Clinical notes routinely attributed deaths to "inherent constitutional weakness" or "primitive susceptibility," completely erasing the documented reality of freezing temperatures, sub-standard rations, and forced labor that directly caused the fatalities.

The Long Road to Historical Reckoning

For decades, the names, medical histories, and final resting places of those who died in the human exhibition circuit remained buried beneath layers of institutional denial and deliberate bureaucratic erasure. It is only through rigorous modern archival recovery, descendant advocacy, and international repatriation movements that these histories have been brought to light.

Reclaiming Identity: Modern historians, forensic researchers, and indigenous community coalitions continue the painstaking work of unearthing municipal health logs, camp medical records, and museum inventories to restore names and dignity to the forgotten dead. The recovery of registers from events like the Tervuren colonial exhibition and the St. Louis World's Fair ensures that the victims are no longer treated as anonymous data points.

The Ongoing Repatriation Struggle: Today, descendant communities and sovereign nations maintain active legal and moral campaigns to secure the repatriation of ancestral remains still housed in university vaults and museum basements. Returning these individuals to their native soils represents a vital step toward correcting the profound medical, ethical, and human rights violations that defined the global human exhibition era.

The Global Aftershocks of Exhibition Pathology

The systemic medical exploitation and institutionalized neglect documented across the major exposition sites of the 19th and 20th centuries were not isolated historical anomalies; they formed a connected, global network of biopolitical control. To fully grasp the enduring magnitude of this chapter, one must examine how these practices permanently altered public health policies, colonial medicine, and the ethical boundaries of human treatment on an international scale.

The Convergence of Colonial Medicine and Exhibition Camps

The medical practices perfected within the fenced compounds of world fairs and human zoos did not stay confined to the fairgrounds. They directly informed and mirrored the methods used by imperial health officers in overseas colonies:

The Standardization of Coercive Health Measures: The tactics used by exposition doctors—such as forced quarantines, unconsented vaccinations, and the suppression of traditional healing methods—served as a testing ground for colonial public health policies. Governments realized that the exhibition infrastructure provided a controlled environment to observe how indigenous populations responded to epidemic diseases under stress, insights they subsequently applied to native populations in occupied territories.

The Normalization of Substandard Care: Just as camp accountants calculated the minimal caloric intake required to keep a performer functional, colonial administrations utilized similar metrics for forced laborers in rubber plantations, mining operations, and railway construction projects. The normalization of preventable malnutrition and untreated illness within the exhibition circuit justified systemic medical neglect on a global scale.

The Structural Erasure of Resistance and Agency

Throughout the grueling ordeal of climate shock, infectious disease, and institutionalized medical abuse, the captives subjected to human exhibitions did not passively accept their fate. Historical recovery of camp records reveals continuous, albeit heavily suppressed, acts of resistance:

Medical Non-Compliance and Sabotage: Archival notes from camp infirmaries frequently record instances were performers actively resisted treatment. Patients refused to swallow bitter or toxic Western pharmaceutical compounds, hid traditional herbal remedies smuggled from home, or simply refused to report to camp doctors until their conditions made concealment impossible.

Collective Mutual Aid: Despite being forcibly segregated from their support systems and paired with strangers, captives often formed clandestine solidarity networks within sick tents. Older members pooled their fading energy to comfort the young, share meager food rations, and perform quiet, forbidden death rites for peers who succumbed to the harsh conditions, preserving their humanity against an apparatus designed to strip it away.

The Permanent Stain on Modern Science

The narrative of Chapter 5 stands as a sobering testament to the cost of unchecked scientific arrogance, racial capitalism, and institutional callousness. By transforming human beings into biological exhibits, experimental subjects, and post-mortem commodities, the organizers and scientific collaborators of the human exhibition era crossed ethical boundaries that forever stained the history of modern medicine, anthropology, and public exhibition.

Chapter 6

Bodies Measured, Humanity Ignored

As the anthropometric enterprise within the human exhibition circuit expanded into the 20th century, the physical evaluation of captives became increasingly mechanized and invasive. Anthropologists, anatomists, and physical physicians did not merely observe; they constructed a formidable array of specialized instruments designed to translate living human bodies into static, numerical proof of racial inferiority.

The Caliper and the Craniometer as Instruments of Power

The physical encounters between researchers and exhibited individuals were governed by heavy, cold metallic tools that symbolize the absolute asymmetry of power within the camp perimeters:

The Standardization of Cranial Imperialism: Researchers placed specialized craniometers and spreading calipers directly against the skulls of living men, women, and children. Every contour of the head was measured to calculate the cephalic index—a ratio meant to correlate brain size and shape with innate intelligence and moral capacity. Captives were forced to sit motionless under the pressure of metal arms clamping against their temples, enduring physical discomfort while a crowd of curious spectators or academic onlookers watched the procedure like a theatrical demonstration.

Photometric Grids and Standing Cages: To capture standardized morphological data, researchers utilized anthropometric framing devices—large wooden or iron grids marked with precise centimeter squares. Individuals were forced to stand naked or semi-nude against these vertical coordinate systems, holding specific postures while photographers documented them from frontal, profile, and rear angles. This process reduced living human beings to flat, grid-aligned specimens, stripping away all individual expression, personal history, and cultural identity.

Physiological Testing Apparatuses: Beyond structural measurements, scientists subjected weakened captives to primitive spirometers, dynamometers, and sensory threshold devices. These tools were used to measure lung capacity, grip strength, pain tolerance, and visual acuity. When exhausted performers failed to meet baseline European performance metrics—a predictable result of chronic malnutrition, damp housing, and active disease—researchers recorded these failures as biological proof of evolutionary stagnation rather than the direct physiological consequences of exhibition neglect.

The Erasure of Subjective Voice and Consent

Crucial to this technocratic ritual was the complete silencing of human subjects. The architecture of the testing rooms and exhibition tents was intentionally designed to prevent any reciprocal dialogue or assertion of personal agency:

The Language Barrier as a Weapon: Most measurements and examinations were conducted without the presence of competent interpreters. Researchers shouted instructions, adjusted limbs by force, and manipulated bodies without explanation. When captives displayed anxiety, fear, or physical resistance, their reactions were systematically misinterpreted and documented in clinical logs as stubbornness, emotional volatility, or lack of higher nervous control.

The Performance of Compliance: Because participation in these invasive studies was tied directly to camp survival—refusal often meant the immediate revocation of food rations, shelter privileges, or meager daily wages—captives had no practical means of withholding consent. The scientific data gathered in these tents was therefore built upon a foundation of structural coercion, weaponizing the captives' own vulnerability against them.

The Academic Legitimization of Harm

The data harvested through these intensive physical examinations did not remain isolated inside exhibition tents; it was rapidly published in prestigious anthropological journals, presented at international scientific congresses, and integrated into academic textbooks across Europe and North America:

Feeding the Eugenics Movement: The measurements, photographs, and clinical notes compiled from exhibited groups provided foundational raw data for the burgeoning eugenics and racial hygiene movements of the early 20th century. Pseudoscientific claims regarding human hierarchy were lent an air of empirical authority entirely because they were backed by "rigorous clinical measurements" gathered from living human displays.

Justifying Colonial Violence: By framing indigenous populations as biologically distinct and permanently inferior through these academic studies, governments and colonial syndicates found intellectual justification for land dispossession, forced labor, and systemic human rights violations across global territories. The physical measurements taken inside the fairgrounds thus served as a vital intellectual anchor for imperial domination, proving that the laboratory and the exhibition were two sides of the same coin.

The Photography of Scientific Objectification

In tandem with mechanical calipers and craniometers, photography became one of the most powerful and pervasive tools for reducing human beings to research subjects. Within the human exhibition circuit, the camera lens was weaponized by anthropologists, ethnologists, and eugenicists who sought to create a permanent visual archive of racial categorization.

The Typological Portrait and the Abolition of Identity

Photography inside the encampments was governed by rigid, standardized rules designed to strip the subject of any personal narrative, emotional expression, or cultural context:

The Standardization of Pose: Captives were required to stand or sit in precise, uniform positions against neutral or grid-lined backdrops. Frontal and profile views were captured with mathematical exactness, mirroring the mugshots utilized by late 19th-century penal systems. This deliberate aesthetic choice aligned the indigenous subject with criminality, deviance, and biological inferiority in the public and academic imagination.

The Erasure of Subjectivity: Photographers routinely commanded subjects to maintain blank, unsmiling expressions and to stare fixedly past the camera. Any sign of individuality, warmth, distress, or resistance was corrected by the photographer. The resulting images presented the subjects not as living, feeling people, but as frozen anatomical types intended to represent an entire race or ethnic group.

The Spectacle of Involuntary Nudity: Under the guise of documenting "primitive authenticity" or conducting anatomical surveys, researchers frequently coerced or forced captives to pose semi-nude or completely naked. These photographs were widely circulated in academic journals, postcards, and popular geographic magazines, satisfying a voyeuristic public appetite while reinforcing the total subordination of the human subjects to the gaze of the Western observer.

The Circulation and Commodification of Anthropometric Images

The photographs taken within the exhibition camps did not remain restricted to private academic archives; they became mass-market commodities that amplified the dehumanization of the captives:

Commercial Postcards and Public Consumption: Millions of postcards featuring typological portraits and staged exhibition scenes were printed and sold to fairgoers as souvenirs. Tourists sent these images across the globe, turning the coerced postures and exposing bodies of the captives into household curiosities. This commercial dissemination ensured that the degradation of the individuals extended far beyond the physical boundaries of the fairgrounds.

Lantern Slide Lectures and Academic Touring: Anthropologists and colonial advocates utilized photographic lantern slides in university lecture halls, museum presentations, and international scientific congresses. Projected in large auditoriums, these towering images of measured bodies served as visual "proof" for lectures on racial hierarchy, social Darwinism, and colonial paternalism.

The Permanent Archival Stigma: Decades after the world's fairs and human zoos closed their gates, these photographic collections remained archived in major national museums, universities, and libraries. For descendant communities, these images represent an enduring legacy of institutional theft—capturing ancestors at their moment of absolute vulnerability and freezing them forever as objects of scientific curiosity rather than honored human beings.

The Nursing Field and the Clinical Surveillance of Captives

As the machinery of anthropometric measurement, physical inspection, and photographic objectification operated within the exhibition compounds, the emerging modern nursing profession became inextricably entangled in this system. While nursing in the late 19th and early 20th centuries was theoretically grounded in patient advocacy, holistic comfort, and compassionate care, its application within the human exhibition circuit revealed a profound ethical divergence. Nurses stationed in camp infirmaries and auxiliary field tents found themselves acting less as advocates for the sick and more as front-line enforcers of institutional control and clinical surveillance.

The Nursing Role as an Instrument of Biopolitical Management

In the structured environment of human zoos and colonial expositions, nurses were tasked with daily oversight of the captives' bodies, transforming routine nursing care into a mechanism of biological monitoring and containment:

The Daily Physical Audit: Camp nurses conducted mandatory morning check-ins and hygiene inspections, recording vital signs, weight fluctuations, and skin conditions not to ensure recovery, but to determine whether a captive was fit for public exhibition. Nurses maintained meticulous logs that fed directly into the statistical models used by physical anthropologists and eugenicists, bridging the gap between clinical observation and racial theory.

Enforcing Compliance with Medical and Administrative Directives: Because nurses were the primary point of daily contact for sick performers, they were responsible for administering the harsh pharmaceutical palliatives, toxic heavy-metal purges, and bitter tonics prescribed by camp physicians. When captives resisted taking unpalatable medicines or protested invasive treatments, nurses often enforced compliance under the threat of reporting them to exposition management, which could result in docked rations or forced stage appearances.

The Normalization of Detachment: Nursing training during this era increasingly emphasized scientific objectivity, clinical detachment, and institutional loyalty. Within the exhibition camps, this professional ethos was pushed to an extreme: nurses were conditioned to view the profound trauma, cultural alienation, and rapid physical waste of the captives as clinical data points rather than human tragedies requiring empathy and intervention.

The Erasure of Holistic Healing and Indigenous Caregiving

The integration of Western nursing protocols into the camps served to systematically displace and pathologize traditional caregiving practices brought by the indigenous participants:

The Criminalization of Traditional Nursing: When female elders or traditional healers among the captive groups attempted to nurse their sick family members using ancestral herbal remedies, poultices, or comforting rituals, camp nurses frequently intervened to confiscate these supplies. Traditional caregiving was labeled as unhygienic, insubordinate, or superstitious, effectively stripping the community of its internal social safety nets.

Imposing Western Hygiene as Cultural Control: Camp nurses enforced rigid European sanitation rules that were often culturally alienating and physically impractical within the improvised, drafty exhibition huts. These rules were rarely designed to improve health; rather, they functioned as disciplinary tools to enforce behavioral conformity and reinforce the ideological narrative of European cleanliness versus native "savagery."

The Long-Term Professional Legacy

The participation of nurses in the biopolitical machinery of human exhibitions left an unacknowledged footprint on the history of the profession. It exposed a dangerous vulnerability within nursing ethics: when professional loyalty is shifted away from the individual patient and toward institutional, corporate, or state objectives, the fundamental duty of care is compromised. The clinical surveillance practiced by nurses in the exhibition camps demonstrated how the tools of healing could be subverted into instruments of measurement, objectification, and control.

The Nursing Field, Resistance, and Ethical Betrayal

The entanglement of the nursing profession within the human exhibition circuit exposed a deep internal crisis between the rhetoric of compassionate care and the reality of institutional compliance. As nurses maintained daily contact with the captive populations, their clinical duties continually intersected with the broader political and scientific goals of exposition management, forcing a complex dynamic of surveillance, suppressed empathy, and occasional covert resistance.

The Paradox of Care Under Duress

Camp nurses occupied an ambiguous position within the exhibition hierarchy. Positioned between the physicians who prescribed harsh pharmaceutical treatments and the administrators who demanded uninterrupted public performances, nurses bore the day-to-day burden of managing human physical breakdown:

Managing Wasting and Epidemics at the Bedside: In makeshift camp infirmaries filled with patients suffering from advanced tuberculosis, measles, or severe frostbite, nurses performed grueling physical labor. They changed bandages, cleaned bedding, and monitored fevers under conditions of extreme supply shortages and administrative indifference. Yet, this labor was rarely directed toward long-term recovery; instead, it was treated as a maintenance operation designed to stabilize patients just enough to return them to the exhibition circuit or quietly process them out before mortality statistics drew public scrutiny.

The Clinical Gaze as a Tool of Classification: Nursing documentation—shift reports, temperature charts, and dietary logs—frequently doubled as observational data for visiting anthropologists and medical researchers. Nurses recorded not only physical symptoms but also behavioral responses, compliance levels, and emotional states. This information was routinely shared with academic investigators, turning the bedside chart into an instrument of racial classification and psychological profiling.

Covert Compassion and Subversive Nursing Acts

Despite the rigid disciplinary framework and the institutional pressure to maintain clinical detachment, archival records and historical studies of camp infirmaries indicate that absolute conformity was not universal. Individual nurses occasionally navigated the strict boundaries of their roles to offer small acts of humanity:

Mitigating Suffering Beyond Orders: In clandestine moments away from the watchful eyes of exposition inspectors and security guards, some nurses provided extra blankets, smuggled nourishing food from staff kitchens to starving captives, or allowed traditional healers brief, unsupervised access to their sick family members. These acts of mercy, though risky, represented quiet rejections of the cold bureaucratic callousness mandated by the fair organizers.

Whispers of Dissent: Certain nursing accounts, preserved in private journals or retrospective memoirs, reveal moments of acute moral dissonance. Nurses wrestling with the realities of children suffering from climate shock or adults dying far from home recorded profound discomfort with the spectacle taking place just outside their tent walls. These private confessions highlight the psychological toll placed on medical staff who were forced to witness the human cost of the enterprise exhibition while remaining bound to an exploitative system.

The Crucial Lesson for Modern Nursing Ethics

The history of nursing involvement in human exhibitions serves as a stark, enduring warning for modern healthcare ethics. It underscores the vital necessity of professional autonomy and unwavering patient advocacy:

The Dangers of Institutional Alignment: When nurses prioritize administrative schedules, institutional reputation, or political ideologies over the physical and emotional welfare of the patient, the core ethical foundation of nursing is fractured.

The Mandate for Cultural Competency: The suppression of indigenous healing traditions by early camp nurses illustrates the historical harm caused by medical ethnocentrism. Modern nursing has since had to confront this legacy, evolving toward culturally safe care that respects diverse traditions, honors patient autonomy, and resists the temptation to pathologize differences.

The Institutional Nursing Apparatus and Historical Anonymity

When examining the specific personnel who staffed the infirmaries, isolation tents, and medical annexes of human exhibitions, colonial expositions, and ethnological displays, a profound historical barrier emerges. Unlike prominent colonial physicians, exposition organizers, or physical anthropologists whose names filled institutional ledgers, academic journals, and government reports, individual nurses working within these camp medical posts were largely rendered anonymous administrative agents.

The Structural Anonymity of Camp Nurses

The systematic lack of named nursing personalities directly tied to the daily care of exhibited captives is a product of how these environments were historically administered:

Subservience to the Medical Hierarchy: In late 19th- and early 20th-century institutional settings, nursing was heavily subordinated to medical authority. Camp infirmaries were directed by exposition-appointed physicians or military surgeons who maintained sole ownership of clinical records, correspondence, and official reports. Nurses executed orders, managed beds, and recorded vital statistics, but their individual identities were routinely swallowed by institutional bureaucracy.

The Erasure of Personnel Records: Archival collections from major world's fairs (such as the Tervuren colonial exhibitions, the St. Louis World's Fair, or the Paris Universal Expositions) typically preserved the names of chief medical officers, directors, and sanitation inspectors while listing nursing staff anonymously as aggregate categories—such as "camp attendants," "red cross detachments," or "infirmary sisters."

Colonial Nursing Corps and Rotational Deployments: Many of the nurses deployed to colonial expositions or overseas imperial displays belonged to official bodies like the Colonial Nursing Association (founded in Britain in 1896) or various military nursing reserves. These nurses were rotated frequently between colonial hospitals, military field units, and temporary exhibition sites, treating their service at exposition camps as brief, routine operational postings rather than defining career events.

The Parallels to Colonial Nursing Figures

While specific biographical accounts of named nurses stationed exclusively inside a human zoo's quarantine tent remain scarce due to historical record-keeping practices, the broader archetype is well-documented through the lens of colonial nursing history:

The Missionary and Imperial Nurse: Figures trained under the Nightingale model who traveled to the colonies or staffed imperial expositions operated under a deeply ingrained ideological framework. They viewed their presence as part of a "civilizing mission," bringing Western hygiene and clinical order to populations they had been taught to view as primitive. This mindset explains why nurses in exhibition camps could simultaneously work long hours tending to sick captives while failing to challenge the fundamental inhumanity of the exhibition system itself.

Institutional Silence: The absence of celebrated nursing personalities stepping forward to expose the horrors of human exhibitions underscores the totalizing power of these environments. Nurses who experienced moral injury or distress—witnessing children succumb to measles, adults waste away from malnutrition, and bodies handed over to university anatomists—kept their grief confined to private, unarchived spaces, constrained by professional codes of obedience and institutional loyalty.

The Epistemological Violence of Clinical Record-Keeping

Beyond the physical instruments of calipers, photographic grids, and pharmaceutical stocks, the daily paperwork generated by nurses, attendants, and camp physicians formed the ultimate documentary weapon of the exhibition era. This record-keeping system did not merely logged health outcomes; it actively constructed the pseudoscientific narrative that justified the subjugation, measurement, and post-mortem commodification of human beings.

The Architecture of the Clinical Chart as a Tool of Reduction

In the camp infirmaries, the nursing chart and the physician's intake log served as bureaucratic engines designed to strip away individual humanity and rebuild the captive subject as a specimen:

The Categorization of Bodies over Persons: Clinical forms were engineered with strict checkboxes and pre-determined diagnostic categories that left no room for individual narrative, personal history, or emotional expression. A captive's name was frequently reduced to an identification number, a tent assignment, or an ethnic designation. Symptoms of profound trauma, grief, and homesickness were systematically translated into cold medical jargon, transforming human suffering into dispassionate data points for institutional archives.

The Weaponization of Diagnostic Language: Medical notes routinely utilized language that pathologized normal human variations and cultural practices. Descriptions of traditional clothing, dietary preferences, or spiritual expressions were annotated as evidence of "backwardness" or "mental inertia." This documentation provided academic researchers with a veneer of objective, clinical authority when they published papers claiming to prove the biological inferiority of the exhibited populations.

Complicity Through Documentation: By meticulously recording temperature spikes, weight loss, and physical decline without intervening with compassionate or adequate therapeutics, nursing and medical logs documented the progressive wasting of human lives as passive observers. These records trace a chilling administrative trajectory: from initial physical measurement upon arrival, to clinical monitoring during decline, to the final administrative sign-off before the body was transferred to a university anatomy department.

The Legacy of Erasure in Historical Archives

The ultimate triumph of this clinical and bureaucratic apparatus was the near-total erasure of the captives' voices from the historical record. When modern historians, ethicists, and descendant communities examine the archives of world's fairs and human exhibitions, they are forced to read through a wall of hostile documentation written by the very individuals who profited from their exploitation.

The Silence of the Subject: Rarely do these historical records capture the perspective, voice, or protest of the person lying on the infirmary cot. The charts record what the nurse observed, what the physician diagnosed, and what the anthropologist measured, but they remain utterly silent on what the human being felt, feared, or desired.

Unmasking the Clinical Gaze: Recognizing how the nursing and medical apparatus functioned within the exhibition circuit forces a critical re-evaluation of early scientific and clinical documentation. It reveals that the tools of healthcare—designed to heal and comfort—were systematically corrupted by a framework of racial capitalism and institutional indifference, transforming the hospital tent into an antechamber for the laboratory and the museum vault.

The Post-Mortem Autopsy as the Final Scientific Extraction

The continuum of measurement, clinical surveillance, and institutional objectification reached its ultimate, grim conclusion upon the death of a captive. When the combination of climate shock, infectious disease, malnutrition, and physiological exhaustion finally broke a human body, the camp infirmary seamlessly transitioned into an anatomical harvesting station. In this final stage, the boundaries between clinical care, anthropometric research, and grave robbing dissolved entirely.

The Transition from Patient to Anatomical Specimen

In the closing hours of a captive's life, the medical staff, including camp physicians and attending nurses, frequently shifted their focus from palliative comfort to prospective anatomical salvage:

The Expedited Death Notification: Archival logs reveal that the moment a patient succumbed to tuberculosis, pneumonia, or dysentery, the administrative protocol bypassed any traditional mourning period or family notification. Instead, the priority was immediate notification of university anatomy departments, craniometric societies, and physical anthropology institutes that held standing claims on the deceased.

The Autopsy as Scientific Harvest: While hospital autopsies are theoretically performed to determine the exact cause of death for clinical clarity, post-mortem examinations within the exhibition circuit functioned as systematic body-part extraction procedures. Physicians meticulously dissected organs preserved brains in formaldehyde and stripped soft tissues to measure muscle density and nerve configurations, seeking biological "proof" of racial hierarchy inside the deceased's internal organs.

The Institutional Pipeline to Museum Vaults: Once the anatomical dissection was complete, skeletons were boiled, bleached, and cataloged with an identification number matching the anthropometric measurements taken when the individual was first forced onto the exhibition grounds. These remains were then shipped to university basements, natural history museums, and anthropological institutes across Europe and North America, where they remained displayed or boxed away for decades.

The Ultimate Denial of Human Dignity

This final industrial-scale processing of human remains represented the ultimate expression of the exhibition era's underlying pathology. By reducing living human beings to measurable data points and subsequently turning their deceased bodies into biological commodities, the architects of human zoos completed a total cycle of commodification.

The nursing charts, anthropometric tables, photographic archives, and anatomical catalogs together formed an unbreakable chain of epistemological and physical violence. They ensured that the captives were denied dignity not only in life—through forced labor, public humiliation, and systematic medical neglect—but also in death, where their very bones were weaponized against their humanity and their descendants.

The Illusion of Holistic Nursing and the Institutionalized Failure of Care

In theory, holistic nursing philosophy emphasizes the integration of physical, emotional, cultural, and environmental dimensions of human health. Yet, within the biopolitical architecture of world fairs, human zoos, and colonial displays, true holistic care was structurally impossible. The institutional framework systematically forced nurses to abandon holistic principles in favor of clinical reductionism, racial categorization, and administrative containment.

The Distortion of Environmental and Cultural Care

Holistic nursing recognizes that an individual's health is inextricably bound to their cultural environment, emotional security, and social community. In the exhibition camps, however, every pillar of holistic wellbeing was actively dismantled by the operational design of the displays:

Pathologizing Cultural Environment: Traditional healing practices, communal grieving, and ancestral spiritual care were not integrated into camp nursing models; instead, they were actively suppressed. Nurses trained in Western sanitation protocols viewed indigenous caregiving as unhygienic or superstitious. By stripping captives of their familiar foods, languages, and healing rituals, nurses enforced an environment of profound psychological isolation that directly aggravated physical waste and disease.

Ignoring the Social Determinants of Health: True holistic intervention addresses the root causes of illness—such as inadequate shelter, freezing temperatures, malnutrition, and exhaustion. Camp nurses, however, were powerless or unwilling to alter the structural conditions of the exhibitions. Rather than advocating for warmer quarters, adequate caloric intake, or an end to forced public performances, nurses treated only the downstream symptoms of systemic abuse, rendering their care fundamentally superficial.

The Failure of Emotional and Psychological Support

Holistic care demands addressing the deep psychological trauma of forced displacement, public humiliation, and constant surveillance. Within the camp infirmaries, emotional support was largely absent:

The Standardization of Emotional Suppression: Captives suffering from acute depression, anxiety, or catatonic withdrawal—manifestations of severe cultural shock and trauma—received no compassionate psychological intervention. Instead, nurses and camp physicians recorded these mental states as biological evidence of racial inferiority or emotional volatility.

Complicity in the Gaze: Because nurses were embedded in the administrative apparatus that managed the public spectacle, they became part of the surveillance state. Their presence in the medical tents did not provide a safe sanctuary from the relentless objectification happening outside; rather, the infirmary was simply another station where the captive's body was measured, charted, and judged.

The Legacy of the Nursing Paradigm Shift

The inability of the nursing profession to apply a genuinely holistic, culturally safe, and human-rights-centered approach during the human exhibition era left a lasting scar on medical history. It exposed how easily nursing ethics can be co-opted by state power, racial capitalism, and institutional convenience.

This historical failure ultimately became a vital catalyst for modern nursing ethics. Today, the nursing profession actively works to undo that legacy through rigorous frameworks of cultural safety, trauma-informed care, and uncompromising patient advocacy—ensuring that the historical tragedy of reducing human beings to measured objects is never repeated in healthcare spaces.

The Post-Exhibition Reckoning and the Evolution of Clinical Ethics

The closure of the last major human exhibitions and colonial displays in the mid-20th century did not automatically dismantle the intellectual and clinical frameworks that sustained them. Instead, the transition from explicit human zoos to post-colonial medical and anthropological practices left a persistent shadow over healthcare and research institutions. Confronting this legacy requires a rigorous examination of how the nursing and medical fields gradually confronted—and continue to reckon with—their historical complicity in institutionalized objectification.

The Long Transition Toward Ethical Accountability

For decades following the dismantling of the global exposition circuit, the medical and nursing professions largely glossed over their active participation in anthropometric measuring, clinical surveillance, and anatomical harvesting. The official histories of nursing and medicine tended to celebrate technological progress and scientific discovery while burying the ethical violations committed within camp infirmaries and university laboratories:

The Awakening of Bioethics: It was not until the post-World War II establishment of international bioethical frameworks—such as the Nuremberg Code and later declarations on human subject's research—that the global medical community began to formally recognize the dangers of unconsented experimentation, anthropometric coercion, and the reduction of human beings to biological specimens. However, these codes initially focused primarily on clinical trials, taking much longer to retroactively address the systemic exploitation of indigenous and colonized populations during the exhibition era.

Re-evaluating the "Clinical Gaze": Modern nursing theory underwent a radical paradigm shift in the late 20th century, moving away from strict technocratic detachment toward frameworks rooted in humanism, empathy, and patient advocacy. Scholars and nurse historians began dissecting how historical nursing practices had been co-opted by state power and racial capitalism, using these dark lessons to teach nursing students the critical importance of questioning institutional orders that compromise human dignity.

Modern Nursing and the Imperative of Cultural Safety

Today, the echoes of the historical failures documented directly inform contemporary nursing education and clinical practice. The total disregard for cultural identity, traditional caregiving, and psychological trauma that characterized camp infirmaries has been systematically countered by modern standards:

From Cultural Competence to Cultural Safety: Modern nursing education has moved beyond superficial "cultural competence" toward cultural safety—a framework originally developed by indigenous nursing leaders (notably in New Zealand). Cultural safety requires healthcare providers to critically examine their own power privileges, institutional biases, and historical legacies of oppression to ensure that marginalized patients receive care that is free of judgment, coercion, and ethnocentrism.

Trauma-Informed Care as an Ethical Shield:

Recognizing that historical and institutional trauma leaves deep physical and psychological scars, modern nursing champions trauma-informed care. This approach ensures that every clinical interaction prioritizes safety, transparency, collaboration, and empowerment—directly inverting the oppressive, non-consensual measuring and charting practices that defined the human exhibition era.

Remembering the Human Beyond the Data

The painful history stands as an enduring reminder that the tools of healthcare—charts, scales, examinations, and clinical observations—are never neutral. When stripped of empathy, respect, and uncompromising dedication to human dignity, clinical practices can easily transform into instruments of surveillance, commodification, and control.

By unearthing the realities of how bodies were measured, and humanity was ignored within the exhibition circuit, contemporary medicine and nursing honor the memory of the victims not merely as data points in an archival ledger, but as whole, complex human beings whose dignity remains a non-negotiable cornerstone of professional ethics.

The Restitution of Dignity and the Ethical Return of the Archive

As contemporary historical recovery and decolonization efforts challenge the long-standing silence of the archives, the focus on Chapter 6's core theme—the violent reduction of human beings to measured objects—has evolved from passive critique into active restitution. Descendant communities, human rights advocates, and progressive medical and academic institutions are systematically confronting the legacy of anthropometric theft and anatomical commodification.

The Movement for Repatriation and Reburial

The physical remains, skeletal collections, and biological samples harvested from human exhibition camps and subsequently locked away in university basements and natural history museums are no longer viewed merely as historical research assets. They are recognized as stolen ancestors whose wrongful imprisonment continues beyond death:

Uncovering Hidden Provenance: Modern provenance research works backward through decades of obfuscated museum catalogs and mislabeled accession numbers. Investigators trace skeletal remains and anatomical artifacts directly back to the specific world's fairs, colonial displays, and exposition camps from which they were seized.

Returning Ancestors to Home Communities: Across the globe, international repatriation efforts have accelerated. Museums and academic bodies are increasingly pressured—and legally mandated—to return ancestral remains to indigenous communities, allowing for formal, culturally appropriate burial rites that restore the dignity, humanity, and sacred peace denied to them by the scientific apparatus of the 19th and 20th centuries.

Redefining Institutional Ethics and Medical Heritage

The painful lessons of anthropometric measurement, clinical surveillance, and the absence of holistic, human-rights-based care within the exhibition circuit are now permanent fixtures in the ethical training of modern healthcare professionals and anthropologists:

Institutional Accountability and Truth-Telling: Leading universities and medical societies are issuing formal apologies for their historical complicity in racial pseudoscience, acknowledging how academic authority was weaponized to legitimize human exploitation. This transparency serves as a vital safeguard against repeating past abuses under new guises.

Embedding Human Dignity at the Core of Practice: By confronting the historical reality where patients and subjects were viewed merely as data points, modern medicine and nursing reinforce the absolute primacy of informed consent, bodily autonomy, and cultural safety. The memory of those measured and ignored in the camp tents stands as a permanent reminder that science and healthcare must always serve human dignity, never erode it.

The Pedagogical Imperative in Modern Healthcare

The journey from the camp tents of the 19th-century exposition circuit to contemporary clinical spaces represents a profound paradigm shift in how the medical and nursing professions understand their ethical obligations. To ensure that the history of anthropometric exploitation, clinical surveillance, and institutionalized dehumanization is never forgotten, modern health science education has integrated these dark chapters directly into its core curricula.

Integrating Historical Trauma into Health Education

Medical and nursing schools increasingly recognize that technical competence alone is insufficient without a deep grounding in historical and social accountability:

Teaching the Roots of Medical Bias: Contemporary curricula examine how early scientific theories—born in the laboratories and exhibition camps of the colonial era—shaped institutional biases that still affect healthcare delivery today. By studying how physical measurements and clinical charts were once weaponized to justify racial hierarchies, students learn to recognize the subtle ways systemic prejudice can manifest in modern diagnostic and treatment frameworks.

Deconstructing the Power Dynamic: Nursing and medical students are taught to critically analyze the inherent power imbalance between healthcare provider and patient. The historical archetype of the camp nurse or physician viewed the captive through a lens of clinical detachment and institutional loyalty—serves as a cautionary benchmark against which modern professionals measure their own commitment to patient-centered advocacy.

The Uncompromising Standard of Informed Consent

The absolute lack of bodily autonomy experienced by human exhibition captives has directly shaped the rigorous legal and ethical frameworks governing patient rights today:

Informed Consent as an Inviolable Right: Every protocol surrounding patient participation in clinical care, data collection, and research is built on the hard-won recognition that individuals own their bodies. Coercion, deception, and the commodification of human subjects—hallmarks of the exhibition era—are strictly prohibited by international codes of ethics.

Protecting Vulnerable Populations: Modern institutional review boards and clinical ethics committees maintain heightened vigilance when evaluating care or research involving marginalized, historically exploited, or economically vulnerable populations, ensuring that historical exploitation is met with active structural protection.

The Enduring Legacy of Human Dignity

The exhaustive exploration reveals a stark and enduring truth: the soul of healthcare lies not in the precision of the instrument, the efficiency of the administrative log, or the volume of data harvested, but in the unconditional respect for human dignity.

When bodies were measured and humanity was ignored beneath the canvas tents of the global exhibition circuit, science lost its moral compass. The ongoing reckoning within nursing, medicine, and the broader scientific community ensures that this history remains visible—not as a monument to past cruelty, but as an eternal vigil reminding every practitioner that every patient is a whole human being, never a specimen.

The Eternal Vigilance of Practice

The physical calipers, the clinical logs, the photographic grids, and the cold administration of camp infirmaries were never benign tools of curiosity; they were instruments of subjugation that systematically converted living, breathing human beings into inanimate research material.

The Unbroken Thread from Past to Present

The legacy of the exhibition circuit's medical and anthropometric apparatus leaves an indelible mark on how contemporary healthcare, science, and society must view the human body:

The Guardrail of Professional Conscience: The history of camp nurses and physicians who surrendered their ethical duties to institutional utility serves as a permanent warning. It demonstrates that professional codes are fragile unless actively defended by practitioners who refuse to let clinical detachment eclipse human compassion.

The Sanctity of the Patient: Every vital sign recorded, every medical chart opened, and every treatment administered in modern practice carries the silent weight of this history. It reminds us that the patient is a complex, autonomous individual with a rich personal and cultural history, never a mere data point, never a specimen, and never a subject for exploitation.

A Final Pledge to Dignity

The systematic reduction of people research subjects under the guise of scientific progress remains one of the darkest chapters in the history of human exhibitions. By dragging this history into the light—acknowledging the victims, interrogating the complicity of the medical and nursing fields, and honoring the resilience of descendant communities—we ensure that their humanity, denied to them in life by the architects of the display circuit, is permanently restored and fiercely protected in every healing space we build today.

Chapter 7

The Invisible Wounds

The Architecture of Psychological Violence

While the physical scars of the human exhibition circuit—manifested in malnutrition, epidemic disease, anthropometric measurements, and post-mortem anatomical extraction—were meticulously documented in clinical logs and research archives, the deepest injuries inflicted upon the captives were entirely unmeasured and unrecorded by their captors. Beneath the physical degradation lay an architecture of psychological violence. To be transformed into a living spectacle for Western entertainment and scientific curiosity was to endure a systematic assault on the human psyche, characterized by chronic stress, profound humiliation, enforced social isolation, and the deliberate erasure of identity.

This chapter examines the invisible dimensions of suffering within the global exhibition apparatus. By looking beyond, the physical symptoms recorded by camp nurses and physicians, we confront the profound psychological devastation experienced by men, women, and children who were caged, displayed, and stripped of their autonomy.

The Chronic Neurological and Emotional Toll of Constant Observation

Living inside an exposition camp meant existing in a perpetual state of hyper-vigilance. Unlike prisoners who retreat behind cell walls or find solitude in confinement, exhibited individuals were subjected to uninterrupted public scrutiny for twelve to fourteen hours a day, exposed to the relentless gaze of thousands of visitors.

The Panoptic Prison of the Stage

Captives lived under the unblinking, voyeuristic eye of the modern spectacle. Whether standing in makeshift "native villages," performing staged daily routines on command, or posing for anthropometric photographers and portrait artists, they were never off-stage. This constant exposure triggered a state of chronic, toxic stress—a prolonged flood of cortisol and adrenaline driven by the acute awareness that every movement, expression, and cultural practice was being watched, judged, mocked, or pathologized.

The psychological burden of this panoptic environment cannot be overstated. Modern trauma psychology identifies continuous surveillance and the denial of private sanctuary as primary drivers of psychological disintegration. Captives had no space to retreat where they were free from judgment, curiosity, or hostility.

Hyper-Vigilance and Anticipatory Trauma

The unpredictable nature of the crowds—ranging from curious families to hostile, taunting mobs—forced captives into a permanent state of defensive psychological readiness. Spectators frequently threw objects, mocked cultural attire, shouted racial slurs, or attempted to touch captives without permission as if they were zoo animals.

This environment fostered an acute sense of helplessness and anticipatory trauma. The inability to secure privacy, quiet, or safety eroded emotional resilience, leading to chronic exhaustion, severe sleep deprivation, and complex anxiety disorders. The neurological system of the captives remained locked in a perpetual "fight-or-flight" response, wearing down their internal coping mechanisms and accelerating physical decline through psychosomatic stress pathways.

Humiliation as an Instrument of Domination

Public display was inherently engineered to invert social standing, strip away personal dignity, and reinforce the ideological superiority of the spectator. Humiliation was not an accidental byproduct of human exhibitions; it was a foundational structural mechanism designed to maintain absolute control.

The Weaponization of Shame

Captives were routinely forced to perform rituals, dances, or domestic chores entirely out of their proper cultural context, turning sacred traditions into commercialized parodies. When crowds laughed, pointed, or treated them with condescending amusement, individuals experienced acute psychological humiliation.

To perform one's sacred customs for the entertainment of those who viewed you as subhuman created a profound internal fracture. Captives were forced to compromise their spiritual and cultural integrity daily just to secure basic food rations or appease exposition guards, breeding deep internal guilt, cognitive dissonance, and spiritual distress.

Infantilization and Loss of Agency

Exhibition management, scientific overseers, and camp nurses treated adult men and women as children or primitive's incapable of autonomous thought or emotional depth. Captives were addressed with condescension, managed through strict disciplinary curfews, and denied any control over their daily routines, diet, or personal interactions.

This forced infantilization systematically undermined their self-worth, agency, and psychological stability, reducing proud community leaders, skilled artisans, and mothers into compliant or psychologically withdrawn performers. The stripping of basic choices—such as what to wear, when to sleep, or how to mourn—eroded the captives' sense of self-determination.

Enforced Social Isolation and Cultural Alienation

The psychological trauma of the exhibition camps was deeply compounded by total severance from familiar social networks, linguistic communities, and cultural support structures. Human beings are inherently social creatures whose psychological stability relies on shared language, mutual understanding, and collective rituals of comfort; the exhibition apparatus severed every single one of these lifelines.

The Shattering of Kinship Bonds

Families and community groups were frequently separated across different exposition sites or placed together under environments so hostile that mutual support became nearly impossible. Parents watched helplessly as their children fell ill in unfamiliar climates, unable to provide traditional comfort or secure adequate medical care.

The inability to mourn deaths properly, celebrate births, or share collective grief left individuals emotionally stranded. In many indigenous cultures, death requires specific communal rites to ensure the spirit's peaceful transition; denying these rites within the camp infirmaries inflicted severe spiritual and psychological trauma upon the survivors.

Linguistic and Geographical Exile

Surrounded by crowds speaking foreign languages, consuming unfamiliar and unpalatable foods, and subjected to harsh, alien climates—such as freezing European winters or sweltering North American summers—captives experienced profound homesickness and disorientation. This severe sensory and cultural deprivation frequently induced depressive states characterized by profound apathy, psychological withdrawal, and, in tragic cases, complete cognitive collapse.

When individuals could no longer communicate their pain, find meaning in their daily existence, or connect with anyone who understood their worldview, they fell into profound despair. Camp physicians often misdiagnosed these trauma responses as "melancholia," "nostalgia," or native apathy, entirely missing the reality that the patients were dying of psychological suffocation.

The Erasure of Identity and the Internalization of Loss

The ultimate psychological injury of the human exhibition circuit was the sustained assault on the captive's core sense of identity. To be gazed upon as an anonymous representative of an entire race is to be stripped of individual humanity.

Reduction to a Monolith

By forcing individuals to represent an entire "type" or exhibit designation, the system denied them their unique personal histories, names, talents, and familial roles. A master carver, a respected healer, or a gifted storyteller was reduced on exposition signage to a generic geographic label.

This total erasure of individual identity forced captives to confront a harrowing existential crisis: the realization that to the surrounding world, they did not exist as people, but as surfaces upon which Western fantasies of savagery and colonial mastery were projected.

The Legacy of Unresolved Grief

The psychological wounds of the exhibition camps did not end when the exhibition gates closed or the tents were struck. Survivors who managed to return to their homelands carried invisible scars that rippled across generations.

The trauma of public exhibitions, institutional dehumanization, and cultural dislocation manifested as chronic generational grief, leaving descendant communities to heal from a historical wound that the official archives deliberately chose not to see. Understanding these invisible wounds is essential for modern historical reckoning, proving that the violence of human zoos extended far beyond physical measurement and anatomical extraction into the very soul of those who survived them.

Psychosomatic Breakdown and the Somatization of Despair

When psychological trauma encounters a totalizing environment where emotional expression is forbidden, grief is ignored, and resistance is futile, the human mind often converts unendurable suffering into physical breakdown. Within the camp tents and exhibition enclosures, the boundary between psychological agony and physical illness dissolved entirely, manifesting as deep somatization.

The Body Bearing What the Mind Cannot Articulate

Captives who were denied any vocabulary of complaint, stripped of legal recourse, and subjected to unyielding scrutiny could not process their trauma through verbal protest. Instead, their nervous systems internalized terror, humiliation, and despair:

Psychogenic Illness and Apathy: Camp medical logs frequently noted patients who simply "lost the will to live"—exhibiting profound lethargy, refusal of food, and rapid physical waste in the absence of any definitive acute infection. While camp physicians lazily attributed this to racial weakness or climatic intolerance, these cases represented textbook instances of psychogenic death and severe depressive withdrawal. The mind, overwhelmed by unrelenting trauma, initiated a shutdown sequence.

The Somatization of Homesickness and Grief: Severe homesickness was recognized by early observers as nostalgia or mal de pays, but within the exhibition camps, it operated as a debilitating, fatal affliction. Chronic insomnia, crushing chest pains, psychosomatic paralysis, and gastrointestinal failure were direct physiological consequences of unremitting stress hormones wreaking havoc on bodies already weakened by poor nutrition and harsh weather.

The Psychological Defense Mechanisms of Survival

Despite the overwhelming machinery of degradation, captives were not passive recipients of psychological destruction. To survive the daily indignity of the exhibition circuit, individuals forged intricate internal psychological defense mechanisms, carving out private sanctuaries within a public panopticon.

Internal Disassociation and Compartmentalized Self

To endure hours of standing on display before jeering crowds, many captives learned to deploy profound psychological disassociation:

The Mask of Performance: Captives mastered the art of separating their inner consciousness from their physical bodies on stage. While outward appearances might have satisfied the expectations of the spectators—performing dances, smiling for cameras, or wearing assigned costumes, their internal minds retreated into deeply guarded spaces of memory, prayer, and ancestral connection.

Mental Resilience and Secret Solidarity: In whispered conversations behind canvas flaps at night, away from the guards and exposition managers, captives shared stories, cracked jokes in their native tongues, and maintained cultural continuity. These clandestine moments of mutual affirmation acted as psychological bulwarks against total depersonalization, preserving their human dignity and collective identity against an apparatus designed to obliterate it.

The Intergenerational Transmission of Exhibition Trauma

The psychological devastation of the human exhibition circuit did not end with the closing ceremonies of world fairs or the dismantling of colonial displays. For the survivors who managed to return to their home communities, the invisible wounds of public display, degradation, and cultural displacement were carried inward, rippling across subsequent generations. This phenomenon—long ignored by mainstream historical archives—represents one of the most enduring legacies of the exhibition era.

The Silence of Return and the Burden of Memory

When survivors returned to their homelands, they frequently faced a complex and painful reintegration process:

The Incommunicability of Suffering: The horrors experienced within the exposition camps—the daily public humiliation, the constant panoptic surveillance, the clinical coldness of camp nurses and anthropologists—were often too profound or too shameful to articulate to families back home. Many survivors chose silence, burying their trauma beneath a protective wall of quiet endurance.

Stigmatization and Alienation: Those who returned were sometimes viewed with suspicion or sorrow by their communities.

Having lived in foreign lands, worn foreign costumes under duress, and witnessed the death of kin in sterile or hostile environments, survivors often felt permanently alienated—fitting into neither the Western world that caged them nor the traditional world they had left behind.

Epigenetic and Cultural Transmission of Trauma

Modern psychological and sociological frameworks recognize that severe collective trauma alters family dynamics and social structures across generations:

Parenting Under the Shadow of Terror: Survivors who endured the hyper-vigilance and institutional control of human zoos often passed down hyper-vigilant parenting styles. The constant underlying fear of arbitrary detention, physical vulnerability, and hostile authorities shaped family environments characterized by intense protectiveness, anxiety, and guardedness.

The Intergenerational Echo of Grief: Descendant communities often inherited a deep, unarticulated grief—an intuitive sense that an ancestral wrong had been committed and left unaddressed. This ancestral trauma manifests today in historical grief, fueling modern demands not only for the repatriation of stolen skeletal remains and artifacts, but for the public acknowledgment and psychological validation of the invisible wounds inflicted upon their forebears.

The Pathologizing Gaze and the Distortion of Native Psyches

Within the operational matrix of the human exhibition circuit, the psychological distress experienced by captives was never interpreted by camp administrators, physicians, or visiting scientists as a normal, rational human reaction to abnormal and abusive conditions. Instead, the entire apparatus relied upon a deeply entrenched ideology of racial pathologization, transforming the very trauma it manufactured into "scientific proof" of the subjects' supposed psychological inferiority.

The Inversion of Cause and Effect

When captives exhibited signs of profound depression, acute anxiety, withdrawal, or cognitive fatigue, camp physicians and psychological observers inverted cause and effect:

Blaming the Victim's Biology: Rather than recognizing that symptoms like apathy, emotional withdrawal, or severe homesickness were the direct result of brutal confinement, grueling public performance schedules, climate shock, and cultural isolation, the medical staff attributed these states to innate racial traits. Clinical notes and anthropological journals frequently described the captives as possessing a "lower threshold for nervous strain," a "primitive emotional constitution," or a "childlike inability to cope with civilization."

Pathologizing Resistance and Grief: Outbursts of anger, grief over lost family members, or refusals to participate in humiliating public spectacles were routinely diagnosed as forms of mental instability, stubbornness, or native volatility. This diagnostic weaponization ensured that any expression of human agency or emotional pain was immediately discredited as pathology, stripping the captive of both dignity and the legitimacy of their suffering.

Restoring the Interior Life

The systematic exploration demonstrates that the violence of the human exhibition era cannot be measured solely by mortality rates, nutritional charts, or stolen anatomical remains. The invisible wounds—the relentless stress of the panoptic gaze, the acute sting of public humiliation, the profound disorientation of cultural exile, and the quiet agony of somatized despair—represent the most enduring tragedy of the human zoo apparatus.

By lifting the veil of archival silence and dismantling the historical pathologization of native psyches, contemporary scholarship restores what the exhibition organizers tried so hard to erase: the complex, resilient interior lives of the captives. Recognizing these invisible wounds is a vital step toward complete historical accounting, ensuring that the psychological humanity of the victims is honored, acknowledged, and never forgotten.

The Reclamation of Narrative and the Healing of Historical Memory

As historical research unearths the deeply buried psychological devastation of the human exhibition era, the movement shifts away from institutional pathology toward active historical recovery. Reclaiming the narrative of the invisible wounds is an essential act of justice, transforming silent suffering into shared historical truth and empowering descendant communities to reclaim the dignity denied to their ancestors.

Dismantling the Myth of the Silent Specimen

For over a century, the archive preserved only the perspective of the observer—the anthropologist's notes, the journalist's review, and the showman's ledger. Modern scholarship, guided by descendant voices and critical trauma theory, actively deconstructs this biased record:

Restoring Emotional Agency: Researchers and historians now read against the grain of archival documents. When a historical log describes a captive as "sullen" or "uncooperative," modern analysis reframes this behavior not as primitive recalcitrance, but as deliberate psychological resistance, quiet mourning, and the fierce protection of an inner self that refuses to be fully conquered.

Centering Survivor and Descendant Voices: The recovery movement prioritizes oral histories, family archives, and community-led documentation. By listening to how descendants articulate the long shadow of generational grief, the academic and historical communities validate the emotional reality of what happened inside the camp tents.

The Path Toward Collective Healing

The invisible wounds of the exhibition era—unresolved grief, cultural displacement, and the trauma of public humiliation—cannot be healed through historical analysis alone. They require a concerted effort of public recognition, institutional restitution, and cultural revitalization:

Public Memorialization: Establishing monuments, commemorative plaques, and museum exhibitions dedicated specifically to the human beings who suffered inside the exposition circuit helps drag the invisible wounds into the open air. Public acknowledgment by the nations and institutions that profited from these displays is a crucial step in collective closure.

Cultural Reconnection as Medicine: For many descendant communities, the ultimate answer to the trauma of exhibition is cultural revitalization—teaching ancestral languages, practicing traditional arts, reclaiming sacred ceremonies, and gathering to share stories. This active preservation and celebration of identity serve as a powerful counter-narrative to the historical forces that sought to erase them.

The Eternal Truth of the Interior Life

The architecture of the human exhibition circuit was designed with terrifying efficiency to crush the human spirit, turning living people into objects, data points, and spectacles. Yet, the history of the invisible wounds reveals an equally powerful truth: the human interior life—our capacity for hope, memory, secret solidarity, and emotional endurance—cannot be completely captured, measured, or destroyed.

By shining a light on the psychological torment of constant observation, the sting of public humiliation, and the deep echoes of intergenerational trauma, Chapter 7 honors the whole, complex human beings who survived the unimaginable. Their psychological resilience stands as an enduring testament to a dignity that no exhibition gate could ever lock away.

The Neurobiological Impact of Chronic Public Exhibition

The chronic stress endured by captives was not merely an emotional reaction to an unpleasant situation; it was a profound, systematic alteration of brain chemistry and nervous system function caused by inescapable, sustained trauma.

The Prolonged Flood of Cortisol and Adrenaline

When individuals are placed under observation in environments characterized by hostility, lack of privacy, and loss of control, the human brain's amygdala triggers a constant state of alarm:

The Exhaustion of the Stress Response: In normal circumstances, the "fight-or-flight" response is a short-term survival mechanism designed to handle acute danger. Within the exposition camps, however, this response was activated continuously for weeks, months, or even years. The sustained flooding of cortisol and adrenaline structurally damages the hippocampus—the brain region responsible for memory processing and emotional regulation—leading to severe cognitive fatigue, memory fragmentation, and chronic anxiety disorders.

Sensory Overload and Environmental Despair: Captives were continuously bombarded with foreign noises, flashing camera equipment, hostile jeers, and shifting weather conditions without any safe harbor. This sensory overload prevented the nervous system from ever achieving homeostasis, pushing individuals into a state of learned helplessness and physical-psychological shutdown.

The Gendered Dimensions of Psychological Trauma

The psychological toll of the human exhibition circuit manifested in distinct, intensely gendered ways. Women and children captured or contracted for display experienced forms of psychological violence specifically tailored to exploit patriarchal and colonial power dynamics.

The Weaponization of Modality and Shame for Women

Female captives faced unique psychological vulnerabilities under the gaze of the Western public:

Hyper-Sexualized Voyeurism: Indigenous women were frequently exoticized through a deeply racialized and sexualized lens in promotional materials and live displays. The psychological trauma of being stared at by crowds who viewed them as living embodiments of primitive temptation inflicted profound violations on their sense of bodily integrity and personal modesty.

Motherhood Under the Microscope: Pregnant women and mothers forced to rear infants within the squalid, freezing, or sweltering conditions of exposition camps endured agonizing psychological stress. Watching their children sicken and die while spectators treated their grief as part of the "authentic show" created an unbearable trauma loop—merging maternal instinct with total institutional powerlessness.

The Infantilization of Children

Child captives grew up internalizing a world where their existence was synonymous with performance and curiosity:

Stunted Emotional Development: Growing up inside a human zoo meant children were denied normal socialization, play, education, and familial security. They learned to view humanity through the distorted mirror of the jeering crowd, fostering deep identity confusion, self-hatred, and long-term developmental trauma.

Language, Silence, and the Defense of the Soul

Language is the primary vehicle through which human beings process trauma, construct shared reality, and seek comfort. Within the exhibition circuit, language was weaponized or suppressed, forcing captives to discover alternative ways to protect their sanity.

The Isolation of Linguistic Exile

Many exhibits grouped individuals from different language groups together under the false administrative assumption that all "natives" of a given continent were interchangeable:

The Terror of Incommunicability: Being unable to speak to anyone in one's native tongue—surrounded instead by guards shouting orders and crowds chattering in foreign languages—created an intense psychological prison. The inability to articulate pain, share memories, or vent frustration trapped suffering entirely inside the individual's mind, accelerating emotional exhaustion.

Secret Codification and Whispers: To combat this isolation, survivors utilized whispered phrases, songs, and non-verbal gestures when overseers were not looking. These acts of linguistic preservation were vital acts of psychological defiance, keeping the home world alive inside a system designed to obliterate it.

The Medical Gaze as Psychological Torture

The presence of physicians, anthropologists, and medical students inside the exposition camps added an insidious layer of psychological terror to the physical degradation.

The Clinical Objectification of the Living Subject

To be measured, poked, and photographed by men in white coats carrying scientific instruments was to be stripped of all humanity:

Dehumanization Through Measurement: When a scientist measured a captive's skull, recorded skin pigmentation, or cast plaster molds of their face while treating them as an inanimate specimen, the psychological impact was profound. It communicated a clear, inescapable message: You are not a person; you are data.

The Fear of the Post-Mortem Horizon: Many captives lived with the terrifying knowledge that their bodies would not even find peace in death. Knowing that academic institutions actively coveted their skeletons for museum vaults created a haunting existential dread, turning the camp infirmary into a place of ultimate psychological terror where medical care was indistinguishable from anatomical predation.

Reconstructing the Internal Geography of Resistance

Despite the overwhelming forces of surveillance, humiliation, and institutional control, the interior geography of the captive's mind remained an unconquered territory.

The Inner Sanctuary of Memory

While exposition managers controlled the physical body on stage, they could not access the internal landscape of memory, storytelling, and spiritual faith:

Mental Relocation: Captives mentally transported themselves back to their homeland recalling the smell of rain on familiar soil, the sound of rivers, the faces of elderly people, and the structure of their home communities. This internal mental migration served as an essential psychological shield, insulating the core self from the degrading reality of the camp.

Collective Resilience and Silent Solidarity: The shared understanding among captives that they were enduring a collective injustice forged profound bonds of solidarity. Even in silence, shared glances of recognition and mutual acknowledgment sustained their emotional endurance, proving that the human spirit could survive even the most calculated systems of erasure.

The Long Shadow of Archival Silence
and the Burden of Proof

The journey toward understanding the invisible wounds of the human exhibition circuit is hindered not only by the severity of the original trauma, but by the structural hostility of the archives themselves. For generations, the burden of proof rested heavily on the victims and their descendants, who were forced to substantiate injuries that the institutional architects of the displays deliberately omitted from official records.

The Absence of Institutional Testimony

Because camp administrators, exposition syndicates, and scientific observers had a vested financial and ideological interest in masking the psychological devastation of their enterprises, the official paper trail is fundamentally silent on matters of mental anguish:

The Erasure of Despair from the Ledger: While ledgers meticulously tracked ticket sales, shipping costs, and nutritional expenditures down to the penny, they contained no columns for grief, nervous exhaustion, or psychological collapse. When a captive suffered a mental breakdown or died of psychogenic withdrawal, the event was either omitted entirely or reframed as a preexisting physical illness or natural mortality.

The Complicity of Journalistic Accounts: Contemporary press reviews and promotional pamphlets frequently described the displayed populations as "happy," "docile," or "curiously amused" by their strange surroundings. This manufactured narrative served to soothe the conscience of the paying public, projecting a false image of contentment that actively gaslit the captives and invalidated their lived reality.

The Restoration of Emotional Truth Through Critical Archival Practice

Overcoming the deliberate sanitization of the historical record requires modern historians, trauma specialists, and descendant researchers to adopt aggressive, empathetic methodologies that read against the grain of traditional colonial archives.

Reading Between the Lines of Administrative Control

To recover the psychological dimensions of the exhibition era, researchers examine ordinary administrative documents through a forensic psychological lens:

Decoding Disciplinary Records: Disciplinary notes detailing "insubordination," "sulking," "refusal to perform," or "stubbornness" are reinterpreted as vital records of psychological resistance and emotional preservation. These reports prove that captives consistently pushed back against their dehumanization, protecting their internal agency even under severe threat of punishment.

Corroborating Private Accounts: The emotional truth of the camps is increasingly illuminated by cross-referencing official records with private journals written by sympathetic foreign observers, secret correspondence from progressive journalists, and diplomatic dispatches that bypassed exposition propaganda. These external perspectives corroborate the acute psychological strain and despair that the official syndicates tried to conceal.

The Unbroken Continuity of Healing

The exploration of the invisible wounds reveals that the legacy of the human exhibition circuit cannot be confined to the physical spaces of the 19th- and 20th-century fairgrounds. The psychological trauma rippled outward across generations, altering family structures, parenting dynamics, and cultural identities within descendant communities.

Yet, alongside this profound generational grief exists an equally powerful narrative of survival and recovery. By dragging the psychological violence of the exhibition camps into the light of historical consciousness, contemporary scholarship validates the suffering of the ancestors and honors their unyielding resilience. The invisible wounds, once hidden beneath a century of archival silence, are finally being acknowledged, mourned, and healed—restoring complete psychological dignity to those who endured the ultimate spectacle of human commodification.

The Cumulative Legacy of Unrecorded Suffering

The Permanent Imprint on Historical Consciousness

The invisible wounds of the exhibition ranging from acute situational trauma and somatized despair to generational grief and the pathologizing gaze of colonial science—form a critical bridge to our modern understanding of historical trauma:

The Refusal of Oblivion: By methodically uncovering the psychological mechanisms of degradation and the quiet, fierce mechanisms of internal resistance, historians and descendant communities ensure that the victims are remembered not merely as statistics of mortality or subjects of anthropometric measurement, but as whole, feeling human beings.

The Healing Imperative: Acknowledging these invisible wounds is not an exercise in passive mourning; it is an active moral imperative. It establishes that the violence of the human exhibition circuit inflicted profound injury upon the human psyche—injuries that required, and continue to require, intentional pathways toward historical truth, public validation, and cultural restoration.

The Sanctuary of the Unconquered Soul

Across every exposition camp, behind every canvas flap, and under the unblinking glare of millions of spectators, captives maintained an invisible, inviolable sanctuary. They remembered their homes, whispered their native languages in secret, mourned their dead in silence, and protected their core identities against a global machinery designed to erase them.

The invisible wounds are real, deep, and generational; yet beside them stands the enduring truth that human dignity, once felt and remembered, can never be completely caged.

The Architecture of Testimony and the Counter-Archive of the Mind

When forced to stand upon the stages of international expositions, world fairs, and colonial villages, captives developed sophisticated psychological mechanisms to protect their core identities from the voyeuristic gaze of the audience:

The Split Self: Survivors and historical reconstructions indicate that many performers engaged in a deliberate psychological compartmentalization. By treating the physical performance on stage as an external mask—a theatrical costume worn out of sheer necessity for survival—they kept their true emotional, spiritual, and intellectual selves entirely detached from the spectacle. The applause, the jeers, and the cameras were directed only at a fiction; the real person remained safely insulated within an inner sanctuary of memory and heritage.

Clandestine Resistance of the Gaze: Rather than passively absorbing the spectator's gaze, captives frequently subverted it. Accounts from sympathetic observers note instances where performers stared back at the crowds not with submission, but with critical detachment or silent indifference, effectively turning the spectators into the observed. This subtle inversion of the panoptic dynamic disrupted the absolute power balance the exposition managers sought to enforce, preserving an essential core of personal agency.

The Sensory Trauma of Dislocation and Environmental Alienation

The psychological injury of the exhibition circuit was deeply rooted in sensory violence. Human beings rely upon familiar sights, sounds, textures, rhythms, and climates to anchor their emotional equilibrium. The exhibition apparatus systematically stripped away every familiar sensory anchor, plunging captives into an environment of profound alienation.

The Assault of the Alien Sensorium

The daily reality of exposition camps exposed captives to jarring sensory shocks that accelerated psychological fatigue and emotional breakdown:

Auditory and Visual Exhaustion: The continuous roar of massive crowds, the metallic clatter of exposition machinery, the flashing glare of early photography equipment, and the relentless chatter of foreign languages created a ceaseless sensory bombardment. Unlike home environments where natural rhythms dictated the flow of daily life, the exposition environment was loud, chaotic, and artificially accelerated.

Climatic and Dietary Incongruity: Forcing tropical or subtropical populations into the freezing, damp winters of Northern Europe or the harsh, fluctuating climates of North American fairgrounds inflicted profound physiological and psychological stress. Combined with meager, unpalatable, and culturally unfamiliar rations, this severe environmental dislocation induced states of chronic apathy, deep homesickness, and cognitive withdrawal that nineteenth-century observers misdiagnosed as primitive melancholy.

The Reclamation of Individual Personhood from Collective Stereotypes

The ultimate psychological violence of the human zoo was the imposition of a collective, flattening stereotype that denied individual uniqueness. Every person brought to the exhibition circuit possessed a specific name, a distinct personal history, specialized skills, familial roles, and a unique emotional inner life.

Restoring the Specificity of Human Experience

To heal from the historical trauma of the exhibition era, modern scholarship and descendant communities actively dismantle the generic labels assigned by historical showmen:

Resisting Monolithic Erasure: Archival recovery projects work diligently to restore the individual identities of those who were reduced on exposition signs and scientific ledgers to mere regional or racial types. By recovering names, familial linkages, and personal narratives, historians challenge the anonymous categorization that the exhibition apparatus relied upon to justify its exploitation.

Honoring the Complexity of Grief and Survival: Recognizing that captives experienced a full spectrum of complex emotions—ranging from profound despair and strategic compliance to fierce internal resistance and unbreakable community solidarity—shatters the racist tropes of docility or passivity manufactured by the original exhibition promoters.

The Persistent Echo of the Interior Life

The psychological trauma mapped across Chapter 7 demonstrates that the true cost of the human exhibition circuit cannot be tallied in numbers, measurements, or economic balance sheets. It resided in the unmapped, unrecorded interior lives of human beings subjected to systemic degradation, constant surveillance, and cultural exile.

Yet, the history of these invisible wounds is equally a history of profound resilience. By acknowledging the psychological violence of the past and honoring the enduring strength of the human spirit, we ensure that the inner lives of those who suffered are never again silenced, forgotten, or ignored.

The Modern Psychology of Historical Trauma and Reparative Justice

Modern trauma specialists, working alongside descendant communities, have established clear frameworks for understanding how unaddressed historical atrocities manifest in present-day mental health disparities:

The Transmission of Chronic Hyper-Vigilance: Just as captives in the exhibition camps were forced into a perpetual state of defensive readiness to survive hostile crowds and arbitrary camp management, descendants often inherit heightened baseline stress responses. This manifests as chronic anxiety, a pervasive sense of vulnerability, and inherited distrust toward dominant institutional authorities, medical systems, and state archives.

The Grief of Cultural Dislocation: The forced removal of ancestors from their homelands, combined with the deliberate suppression of their languages, spiritual practices, and social structures during exhibitions, created lasting cultural fractures. Descendants frequently experience an unarticulated sense of loss—an ancestral grief stemming from the disruption of traditional knowledge transmission and kinship networks.

Reparative Justice as a Psychological Necessity

Addressing these enduring invisible wounds requires more than academic acknowledgment; it demands active, systemic reparative justice designed to restore dignity and emotional closure to affected communities:

Institutional Apologies and Public Validation: When national governments, scientific institutions, and museum syndicates formally acknowledge their complicity in human exhibitions, it provides a vital psychological validation for descendant communities. Official admissions of guilt help dismantle the lingering remnants of colonial victim-blaming, shifting the burden of shame away from the victims and back onto the institutions responsible.

Community-Led Healing Initiatives: True psychological recovery is anchored in community empowerment. Funding culturally grounded mental health programs, supporting language revitalization projects, and backing community-led initiatives to rebury or honor ancestors whose remains were mishandled during the exhibition era serve as powerful therapeutic acts of collective restoration.

The Ethics of Witnessing and the Responsibility of the Historian

To study the psychological dimensions of the human exhibition circuit is to assume ethical responsibility. Historians, researchers, and writers who engage with the trauma of the past cannot remain neutral observers; they must act as ethical witnesses to a history designed to be forgotten or minimized by its perpetrators.

Overcoming Historical Complicity

For over a century, the dominant historical narrative treated human exhibitions as quaint, misguided curiosities of a bygone era or as benign spectacles of popular entertainment. This sanitization was a deliberate continuation of the violence:

Refusing the Spectator's Perspective: Ethical historical inquiry demands that we deliberately step out of the shoes of the paying spectator peering into the camp enclosure. Instead, scholarship must align itself with the lived reality, emotional vulnerability, and quiet resistance of the captives.

Challenging Archival Erasure: Because the institutional record is inherently biased—built on the ledgers of showmen, the clinical notes of anthropologists, and the sensationalist headlines of colonial newspapers—historians must read against the grain to rescue the interior lives of the victims from deliberate oblivion.

The Unconquerable Humanity of the Displayed

The invisible wounds, the chronic stress, the sharp sting of public humiliation, the profound disorientation of cultural exile, and the quiet agony of somatized despair—were real and devastating. Yet, standing resolutely alongside these injuries is the enduring record of human resilience. Captives maintained their dignity through whispered native phrases, shared glances of solidarity, mental migrations back to their homelands, and the fierce protection of an inner self that refused to be put on display.

By bringing these invisible wounds into the light of historical consciousness, we honor the whole, complex human beings who survived the unimaginable. Their psychological endurance stands as an eternal testament to a truth that no exposition gate, colonial decree, or archival silence could ever lock away: that human dignity, once felt and remembered, remains forever unconquered.

Chapter 8

Who Was Responsible?

The global human exhibition circuit—encompassing world's fairs, colonial expositions, traveling circuses, and ethnographic displays—was not the byproduct of a few isolated opportunists. It was an institutionalized, systemic enterprise sustained by the active participation or tacit consent of entire societal sectors. To understand how human beings could be caged, measured, commodified, and publicly displayed on a mass scale, we must examine the distinct complicity of the various actors who built, maintained, and consumed the apparatus.

Furthermore, by evaluating their actions through the lens of modern standards of medical, scientific, and corporate ethics, we confront a profound historical divergence—measuring the ethical vacuum of the nineteenth and early twentieth centuries against our contemporary frameworks of human rights.

The Complicity of Physicians and Medical Professionals

Physicians and medical researchers occupied a position of immense institutional power within the human exhibition circuit, acting as both administrative gatekeepers and scientific exploiters. Rather than serving as protectors of human health, medical personnel frequently subordinate their ethical duties to the demands of colonial ideology and anthropological curiosity.

The Subversion of the Oath and Clinical Duty

Within the exposition camp infirmaries, the fundamental ethical principle of primum non Nocera (first, do no harm) was systematically inverted. Captives brought to physicians suffering from malnutrition, climate shock, severe depression, or infectious diseases often received substandard care or were treated merely as living diagnostic subjects:

Medical Voyeurism and Pathologization: Physicians routinely documented the physical and psychological decline of captives not because of abusive camp conditions, but as "proof" of biological inferiority. Symptoms of profound trauma, grief, and homesickness were pathologized as native apathy or constitutional weakness.

Complicity in Anthropometric Extraction: Medical officers frequently collaborated with anthropologists to measure bodies, record physiological responses under duress, and extract anatomical specimens. In many tragic instances, physicians monitored dying patients not to alleviate their suffering, but to secure immediate access to their bodies for post-mortem dissection and skull collection upon expiration.

Comparison with Modern Healthcare Ethics

Under modern medical ethics—governed by frameworks such as the World Medical Association's Declaration of Helsinki, the Nuremberg Code, and international standards of informed consent—the conduct of nineteenth-century exhibition physicians represents a catastrophic moral failure:

Informed Consent vs. Coercion: Modern healthcare mandates absolute voluntary consent, free from coercion, exploitation, or power imbalances. Exhibition captives, trapped within totalizing environments without legal agency, were incapable of giving true informed consent.

Duty of Care: Contemporary bioethics dictates that a physician's primary loyalty is strictly to the patient's well-being, superseding state interests, racial ideologies, or scientific ambition. Exhibition physicians routinely violated this primary duty, functioning instead as instruments of state control and commercial exploitation.

Scientists, Anthropologists, and the Weaponization of Science

The academic establishment provided the ideological foundation and intellectual justification for human exhibitions.

Anthropologists, ethnologists, and natural historians viewed the exposition camps as living laboratories, treating human beings as specimens rather than people.

Transforming People into Data Points

Scientists utilized the exhibition circuit to validate theories of racial hierarchy, polygenism, and social Darwinism:

The Spectacle of Measurement: Anthropologists subjected captives to humiliating public and private examinations—recording cranial dimensions, skin pigmentation, body proportions, and dental structures. These measurements were published in prestigious academic journals to "prove" the linear progression of human evolution, placing Western Europeans at the apex and indigenous populations at the base.

The Preservationist Paradox: Scientists often justified the study of displayed populations through a paternalistic sense of urgency, claiming that indigenous groups were "vanishing races" destined to extinction under the pressures of modernity. This narrative masked the reality that the exhibition camps themselves actively accelerated the mortality and physical decline of the captives through disease and neglect.

Comparison with Modern Research Ethics

Modern scientific research is bound by strict institutional review boards (IRBs), human subjects' protection protocols, and ethical principles emphasizing respect for persons, beneficence, and justice:

Respect for Persons: Modern standards require treating all research participants as autonomous agents with inherent dignity. The exhibition era's treatment of living humans as inanimate objects of study violates the core tenets of modern ethical research.

The Rejection of Scientific Racism: Contemporary anthropology and biological sciences explicitly reject the racial typologies and pseudoscientific hierarchies that underpinned the human zoo circuit, recognizing them as ideological tools designed to justify colonialism and enslavement.

Zoo Officials, Showmen, and Corporate Syndicates

The operational architects of the exhibitions—promoters, circus owners, fair directors, and municipal authorities—engineered the commercial machinery of human display. Motivated by profit and civic prestige, they treated human performers as movable property and economic cargo.

The Business of Dehumanization

Showmen like Carl Hagenbeck and corporate fair syndicates transformed the exhibition of foreign peoples into a highly lucrative global industry:

Contractual Deception and Coercion: Promoters relied on predatory contracts, withheld wages, debt bondage, and physical confinement to maintain control over troupes. They actively manipulated public perception through sensationalist advertising, portraying diverse cultures through crude, uniform stereotypes of savagery to maximize ticket sales.

Neglect of Basic Welfare: Profit margins took precedence over human survival. Overcrowded living quarters, inadequate winter clothing, poor sanitation, and restricted diets were standard operational practices designed to minimize overhead costs, directly resulting in preventable outbreaks of disease and high mortality rates.

Comparison with Modern Corporate Ethics

Contemporary business ethics, labor laws, and international human rights standards—such as the International Labour Organization (ILO) conventions and corporate social responsibility (CSR) frameworks—prohibit the practices standard in the human exhibition industry:

Labor Rights and Fair Compensation: Modern labor standards outlaw forced labor, wage withholding, deceptive contracting, and hazardous working conditions.

Human Rights Compliance: Corporations today are held accountable for human rights abuses within their supply chains and business operations. The commercial commodification of human beings practiced by exposition syndicates would today be classified as human trafficking and severe human rights violations.

Government Authorities and Imperial Bureaucracy

Imperial governments, colonial ministries, and municipal authorities were deeply implicated in the human exhibition circuit, providing the political authorization, diplomatic clearance, and logistical infrastructure necessary for their operation.

The State as Enabler and Beneficiary

Governments viewed human exhibitions as vital instruments of imperial propaganda:

Projecting Colonial Power: World's fairs and colonial expositions were heavily subsidized by states eager to showcase colonial conquests, justify imperial expansion to domestic taxpayers, and foster national pride. Displaying colonized subjects as docile, primitive, or exotic served to validate the civilizing mission narrative.

Issuing Permits and Overseeing Logistics: Colonial governors facilitated the recruitment and exportation of indigenous troupes, often utilizing military force, taxation pressure, or bureaucratic coercion to compel communities to supply performers to European and North American promoters.

Comparison with Modern State Responsibility

Under modern international law, state actors are bound by human rights treaties, the United Nations Declaration on the Rights of Indigenous Peoples (UNDRP), and international humanitarian standards:

Protection of Vulnerable Populations: Modern governments bear a legal and moral obligation to protect vulnerable indigenous populations from exploitation, trafficking, and public degradation.

Historical Accountability: Contemporary state ethics increasingly demand institutional reckoning, formal apologies, and reparative justice for past state-sponsored human rights abuses and colonial atrocities.

Missionaries and Religious Institutions

Religious organizations and missionaries maintained a complex, often contradictory relationship with the human exhibition circuit. While some missionary groups occasionally raised ethical concerns regarding the physical welfare of performers, the broader missionary establishment was frequently entangled in the paternalistic ideologies that enabled the exhibitions.

The Ideology of Paternalism and Moral Superiority

Missionaries operated within the same civilizational framework that justified the display of non-Christian peoples:

Cultural Erasure as Salvation: Mainstream missionary efforts often sought to eradicate indigenous spiritualities, languages, and cultural practices, viewing them as primitive or demonic. This ideological stance dovetailed neatly with the exposition narrative that framed displayed peoples as subjects in urgent need of Western uplift.

Silence and Complicity: While individual missionaries occasionally protested the harsh conditions or public degradation of specific troupes, institutional religious bodies largely remained silent, viewing the encounters through a lens of spiritual conversion rather than fundamental human rights.

Comparison with Modern Religious and Humanitarian Ethics

Contemporary religious ethics and global humanitarian organizations have largely moved away from coercive paternalism toward frameworks of interfaith dialogue, cultural respect, and human rights advocacy:

Recognition of Indigenous Dignity: Modern humanitarian ethics emphasize the preservation of indigenous cultural heritage, self-determination, and the protection of vulnerable communities from exploitation, aligning moral authority with social justice rather than colonial domination.

The Public and the Spectator

Ultimately, the human exhibition circuit could not have sustained itself without the enthusiastic participation of millions of ordinary citizens who purchased tickets, crowded the camp enclosures, and consumed the spectacle as entertainment.

The Consumer as an Active Participant

The public was not an innocent or deceived observer; they were active consumers of racialized entertainment:

Consuming the Other: Visitors flocked to expositions to experience the thrill of the exotic, reinforcing their own sense of modernity, civilization, and racial superiority through the degradation of others. The normalization of human display created a cultural consensus that treated non-Western people as natural objects of curiosity.

Complicity Through Silence: Even when witnessing clear signs of distress, illness, or mistreatment among captives, spectators largely accepted the fictional framing provided by showmen, treating human suffering as part of the authentic show.

Comparison with Modern Consumer Ethics

Contemporary consumer ethics places moral responsibility on the end-user, emphasizing ethical consumption, human rights awareness, and the rejection of exploitative entertainment:

Ethical Scrutiny of Entertainment: Modern society increasingly rejects the commodification of human beings in entertainment—condemning human zoos, freak shows, and exploitative media formats. The contemporary public is expected to exercise critical awareness regarding the ethical origins and human costs of the goods and services they consume.

The Structural Web of Responsibility

The human exhibition circuit was sustained not by a single rogue actor, but by a synchronized web of complicity spanning medicine, science, commerce, governance, religion, and public consumption. When measured against modern standards of healthcare ethics, human rights, and scientific integrity, the actions of these historical actors reveal a profound moral bankruptcy. Recognizing this distributed responsibility is essential for historical truth, ensuring that the legacy of the human exhibition era is understood not as a series of unfortunate misjudgments, but as a systemic failure of human empathy and institutional ethics across an entire global society.

The Institutionalization of Indifference and the Legal Frameworks of Impunity

To fully comprehend the depth of responsibility across nineteenth- and twentieth-century societies, we must examine how legal and institutional frameworks actively protected the human exhibition industry from accountability. The perpetrators of these displays operated not in defiance of the law, but frequently under its explicit protection, patronage, and bureaucratic sanctions.

Legal Structures and the Absence of Personhood

The foundational mechanism that allowed human exhibitions to flourish was the systematic denial of legal personhood to the colonized and indigenous populations displayed within them:

Colonial Jurisprudence and Subjugation: Under the legal doctrines of imperial powers—such as the French Indigénat regime or various British colonial statutes—indigenous subjects were categorized as sujets rather than citoyens. This legal status stripped them of habeas corpus, freedom of movement, and labor rights, leaving them entirely at the mercy of administrative decree and commercial contract.

The Legal Fiction of Voluntary Performance: Exhibition contracts were upheld by European and American courts as binding civil agreements, despite being forged under conditions of economic destitution, linguistic deception, and physical isolation. Legal systems recognized the commercial rights of the showmen and syndicates while treating the performers as movable assets or non-entities incapable of seeking judicial redress.

Comparison with Modern International Jurisprudence

When evaluated against modern human rights frameworks, such as the Universal Declaration of Human Rights (UDHR) and international anti-trafficking conventions, the legal protection afforded to human zoos reveals an institutionalized system of state-sanctioned exploitation:

The Prohibition of Human Trafficking and Enslavement: Modern international law criminalizes any system that buys, sells, transports, or holds human beings under conditions of forced labor and public degradation, regardless of contractual paperwork.

Universal Human Rights Protection: Contemporary legal norms establish that fundamental human rights are inalienable; they cannot be signed away by contract, nor can they be revoked by colonial status or citizenship classification.

The Role of Municipal Governments and Civic Boosters

While commercial syndicates and colonial ministries provided the macro-level structure for human exhibitions, municipal governments and local civic boosters were critical local enablers. Mayors, city councils, chambers of commerce, and world fair committees eagerly competed to host ethnographic displays as a measure of civic pride and economic revitalization.

Civic Prestige and the Politics of Display

Local authorities viewed human zoos and colonial villages as major tourist attractions that generated municipal revenue and projected modern urban importance:

Subsidies and Land Grants: City governments frequently provided prime public land—often within urban parks or municipal exhibition grounds—free of charge or at heavily subsidized rates to exhibition promoters. They funded infrastructure, provided police security, and integrated the human camps into official civic celebration schedules.

Sanitation and Public Health Complication: Municipal health boards maintained a selective standard of oversight. While they occasionally inspected camps for overt public health hazards that might threaten the visiting European public, they routinely ignored the chronic malnutrition, psychological deterioration, and high baseline mortality rates of the captives, treating human lives as expendable municipal inventory for the duration of the exposition.

Comparison with Modern Municipal Governance and Public Ethics

Modern municipal governance operates under strict public accountability, urban human rights charters, and ethical guidelines governing the use of public space and civic funds:

Prohibition of Discriminatory Public Displays: Contemporary cities are legally and ethically barred from hosting events that promote racial degradation, human commodification, or cultural exploitation on public property.

Public Welfare Mandates: Modern municipal authorities hold a non-negotiable duty of care to protect all human beings within their jurisdiction, ensuring that public events comply with labor, safety, and human rights standards.

The Mass Media and the Manufacture of Public Consent

The press, publishing houses, and early visual media played a pivotal role in creating and sustaining the demand for human exhibitions. Newspapers, illustrated magazines, promotional postcards, and travelogues served as ideological transmission belts that normalized the dehumanization of displayed populations.

Journalistic Complicity and Sensationalism

The nineteenth- and twentieth-century media industry thrived on sensationalism, actively manufacturing public appetite for exoticized and racialized spectacles:

Promoting Racial Hierarchies: Editorial boards and journalists routinely deployed patronizing, paternalistic, or outright racist language to describe exposition performers, framing them as living relics of human prehistory. This constant media saturation conditioned the reading public to view human beings as natural curiosities rather than peers.

Whitewashing Camp Realities: When deaths, escapes, or severe abuses occurred within the exhibition camps, media outlets either suppressed the stories or framed them through a lens that blamed the victims' biology or cultural background, effectively shielding the promoters and municipal authorities from public backlash.

Comparison with Modern Media Ethics

Contemporary journalism and media production are guided by codes of ethics established by professional organizations, emphasizing accuracy, fairness, human dignity, and the avoidance of harmful stereotypes:

Ethical Reporting Standards: Modern media ethics strictly prohibit the exploitation, dehumanization, or racial stereotyping of vulnerable populations for sensationalism or profit.

Accountability and Truth-Seeking: Contemporary journalistic integrity require independent investigation, giving voice to marginalized subjects, and exposing institutional exploitation rather than acting as a propaganda arm for commercial enterprises.

The Architecture of Collective Accountability

The examination of who was responsible for the human exhibition circuit demonstrates that the phenomenon was an integrated systemic failure across every pillar of Western and colonial societies. Physicians abandoned their oaths, scientists weaponized pseudoscientific racism, corporate syndicates commodified human lives, governments and municipal authorities provided legal and logistical cover, missionaries enforced cultural paternalism, media outlets manufactured consent, and the public consumed the spectacle as casual entertainment.

When measured against modern standards of healthcare ethics, human rights law, corporate responsibility, scientific integrity, and media accountability, the historical actors of the human exhibition era stand condemned by an unbridgeable ethical chasm. Recognizing this comprehensive network of responsibility ensures that the history of human zoos is understood not as an anomaly of bad actors, but as a profound structural indictment of an entire era's moral framework—an accounting that remains vital for contemporary restorative justice and historical truth.

The Institutionalization of Accountability Deficits and Corporate Shields

Continuing our examination of Chapter 8, we turn to how the corporate and bureaucratic structures surrounding human exhibitions systematically insulated organizers, investors, and state actors from legal liability or moral censure when catastrophes occurred within the camps.

The Shield of Bureaucratic Abstraction

The business of displaying human beings was purposefully fragmented across complex corporate hierarchies, third-party talent brokers, independent logistics contractors, and municipal committees:

Diffusion of Responsibility: By dividing the labor of recruitment, transport, exhibition management, and scientific sampling among numerous distinct entities, no single individual or corporation was forced to carry the full weight of accountability. If a performer died of exposure, malnutrition, or medical neglect, blame was easily deflected down the chain of command—attributing the fatality to local acclimatization issues, pre-existing health conditions, or independent contractor negligence rather than systemic corporate design.

The Shield of Commercial Secrecy: Financial ledgers and management logs were treated as proprietary business documents rather than public records. This commercial privacy prevented independent oversight, allowing syndicates to conceal high morbidity and mortality rates behind closed administrative doors while projecting an image of benign cultural education to the paying stockholders.

Comparison with Modern Corporate Liability and Governance

Modern international law, corporate accountability frameworks, and human rights due diligence standards completely reject these historical mechanisms of avoidance:

Non-Delegable Duty of Care: Contemporary corporate governance dictates that organizations cannot contract away their responsibility for human safety and labor rights. Companies operating international events, traveling productions, or supply chains are held legally and financially liable for the well-being of all participants, regardless of intermediaries or subcontractors.

Corporate Transparency and Whistleblower Protections: Modern regulatory bodies require open reporting, independent oversight, and strict compliance with labor and human rights laws, ensuring that corporate secrecy can no longer be used to mask human exploitation or systemic negligence.

The Complicity of Academic Institutions and Museums

The architecture of responsibility for the human exhibition circuit extends deeply into the academic and cultural institutions that collected, studied, and preserved human remains and cultural artifacts acquired during the exhibition era. Universities, natural history museums, and anthropological societies were not neutral observers; they were active financial and intellectual stakeholders in the human zoo enterprise.

The Academic Acquisition Pipeline

Universities and museums frequently partnered directly with exposition syndicates and colonial governments to leverage the camps as supply chains for research collections:

The Commodification of Human Remains: Anthropologists and anatomists routinely arranged to secure the skeletal remains, soft tissue samples, and bodily measurements of performers who died in captivity or whose bodies were exhumed from exhibition camp burial sites. These remains were cataloged and stored in museum basements and academic vaults under pseudoscientific classifications, treating deceased human beings as permanent research specimens.

Institutional Legitimation: By hosting academic conferences in conjunction with world fairs, publishing pseudoscientific papers based on data gathered in human camps, and displaying ethnographic collections acquired through unequal colonial power dynamics, academic institutions provided intellectual respectability to what was fundamentally a system of human exploitation.

Comparison with Modern Museum Ethics and Repatriation Standards

Modern museum governance, governed by international charters, professional codes of ethics (such as the International Council of Museums guidelines), and specific legislation like the Native American Graves Protection and Repatriation Act (NAGPRA) in the United States, stands in stark moral opposition to nineteenth-century academic practices:

Ethical Acquisition and Provenance Research: Contemporary museums are required to conduct rigorous provenance research to ensure that artifacts and human remain in their collections are acquired ethically, with valid consent and clear legal title.

Repatriation and Restitution: Modern standards mandate the unconditional return of stolen human remains, sacred objects, and cultural heritage to descendant communities and native nations, recognizing that scientific inquiry can never supersede basic human dignity and the right to a respectful burial.

The Complicity of Legal and Judicial Systems

Continuing our critical evaluation, we must examine the formal legal and judicial systems that not only permitted the human exhibition circuit to operate but actively enforced its parameters and protected its organizers from judicial interference. Courts, magistrates, and legal theorists provided the structural enforcement mechanism that transformed human beings into legally recognized commodities.

The Judicial Enforcement of Servitude and Confinement

When disputes arose between exhibition managers and performers—such as attempts to break predatory contracts, demands for withheld wages, or intolerable camp conditions, the judiciary consistently sided with commercial and colonial interests:

Enforcing Involuntary Contracts: Judges routinely ruled that performance contracts signed by indigenous individuals or colonial subjects were legally binding civil agreements. They ignored or dismissed evidence of linguistic deception, lack of legal representation, duress, and economic desperation, choosing instead to uphold the sanctity of commercial property and contract law over fundamental human liberty.

The Criminalization of Resistance: When captives attempted to escape their enclosures, strike against unfair treatment, or protest public humiliation, colonial and municipal police forces were deployed to arrest them. Courts prosecuted escaping performers as runaway contract breakers or vagrants, legally returning them to the custody of the showmen and reinforcing absolute institutional control.

Comparison with Modern Judicial Ethics and International Human Rights Law

When measured against contemporary judicial standards and international human rights jurisprudence, the behavior of nineteenth- and twentieth-century courts represents a profound corruption of the rule of law:

The Protection of Fundamental Rights: Modern legal systems operate on the principle that basic human rights—including freedom from forced labor, arbitrary detention, and public degradation—are inalienable and superior to private commercial contracts. No modern court would enforce a contract that commodifies human beings or strips them of bodily autonomy.

Access to Justice and Equal Protection: Contemporary legal frameworks guarantee vulnerable populations the right to independent counsel, habeas corpus, and judicial protection against exploitation, ensuring that courts serve as a shield for human dignity rather than an instrument of corporate and colonial oppression.

Capital Investment in Human Commodification

The logistics of transporting hundreds of performers across oceans, constructing sprawling exposition grounds, and mounting massive marketing campaigns required vast amounts of capital:

Profit from Exploitation: Major commercial banks and private investors eagerly funneled money into exposition syndicates, anticipating high returns driven by massive ticket sales and government subsidies. These financial institutions treated human exhibits as standard commercial commodities, calculating risk and return on investment without regard for the human costs embedded in the supply chain.

Shielding Investors from Moral Inquiry: Financial backers operated behind corporate boards and investment portfolios, insulated from the day-to-day squalor, disease, and psychological distress of the camps. Their capital sustained the physical and administrative infrastructure of the human zoo network, making them silent but indispensable partners in the exploitation.

Comparison with Modern Ethical Investment and Financial Standards

Contemporary financial markets and investment ethics—exemplified by Environmental, Social, and Governance (ESG) criteria, socially responsible investing (SRI), and international finance standards such as the Equator Principles—stand in stark contrast to nineteenth-century capitalist practices:

Mandatory Social and Human Rights Audits: Modern financial institutions are increasingly held accountable for the ethical impact of their investments, requiring rigorous human rights due diligence before funding projects, events, or corporate supply chains.

Rejection of Unethical Commerce: Financial backing for enterprises that commodify human beings, violate labor laws, or exploit vulnerable populations is legally prohibited and socially condemned. Modern investment ethics mandate that capital must serve sustainable, human-centric development rather than profit derived from human degradation.

The Absolute Ethical Failure of an Entire Society

The exhaustive evaluation across this chapter demonstrates that the human exhibition circuit was not an accidental moral lapse, but a fully integrated, financially incentivized, and legally protected enterprise upheld by every major pillar of Western civilization.

Physicians, scientists, corporate showmen, government authorities, municipal boosters, missionaries, media syndicates, legal systems, and financial investors all shared in the construction and maintenance of this global system of human display.

Measured against modern standards of healthcare ethics, human rights law, corporate social responsibility, scientific integrity, and ethical investment, the historical actors of the exhibition era stand indicted by an unbridgeable moral chasm. Recognizing this total societal responsibility is essential for historical truth, ensuring that the human zoo era is understood not as a series of isolated mistakes, but as a profound, systemic failure of human empathy and institutional ethics.

The Global Complicity of International Networks and Transnational Syndicates

The commodification of human beings was not restricted to single nations or domestic empires; it operated through an extensive, highly coordinated international marketplace that crossed borders with total administrative and legal impunity.

The Transnational Traffic of Human Cargo

Exhibition promoters and talent syndicates functioned as multinational corporations avant la letter, establishing agents and booking offices across major global financial capitals:

Cross-Border Talent Brokering: Promoters regularly leased troupes of performers across international borders, transferring groups from German zoological gardens to French world's fairs, British expositions, and American amusement parks. This transnational mobility operated under bilateral trade agreements and colonial transit permits that treated human performers as commercial cargo subject to customs declarations and international shipping manifests.

The Normalization of Extraterritorial Exploitation: When operating abroad, foreign syndicates relied on the host nation's legal and police systems to suppress dissent, prevent desertion, and enforce strict confinement. Host governments willingly extended police protection to foreign showmen, prioritizing international trade prestige and entertainment diplomacy over the basic human rights of the foreign nationals within their borders.

Comparison with Modern International Anti-Trafficking and Human Rights Standards

When measured against modern international law—including the Palermo Protocols on Human Trafficking, international labor conventions, and cross-border human rights enforcement mechanisms—the transnational operations of historical exhibition syndicates represent systemic global criminality:

Prohibition of Cross-Border Exploitative Transit: Modern international jurisprudence strictly outlaws the recruitment, transportation, and harboring of people through deception, coercion, or abuse of power for the purpose of public exploitation.

State Cooperation for Human Protection: Contemporary international agreements mandate that states cooperate to prevent human trafficking, protect vulnerable foreign nationals, and prosecute transnational entities that violate fundamental human rights, completely reversing the nineteenth-century model where states collaborated to facilitate human commodification.

The Complicity of Academic Presses and Educational Publishers

The dissemination of pseudoscientific racism and colonial paternalism relied heavily upon the printed word, academic journals, and school curricula.

The Printing Press as an Instrument of Ideological Standardization:

Academic publishers and textbook authors actively propagated the narratives that justified the public display of non-Western people:

Legitimizing Pseudoscientific Journals: Academic presses eagerly published articles, monographs, and anthropometric studies generated from data collected inside human zoo camps. By binding these racist measurements and observations within the formal covers of peer-reviewed journals and university publications, publishers lent an aura of undeniable scientific authority to what was essentially exploitative voyeurism.

Shaping Early Educational Curricula: School textbooks throughout the late nineteenth and mid-twentieth centuries routinely incorporated descriptions of indigenous populations drawn directly from exposition propaganda and travelogues. Children in Western nations were taught to view diverse cultures through a hierarchical, condescending lens, embedding colonial prejudices deep into the foundational education of successive generations.

Comparison with Modern Academic and Educational Ethics

Modern publishing ethics, peer-review standards, and educational guidelines stand in absolute opposition to the propagation of racial hierarchies and pseudoscientific exploitation:

Commitment to Ethical Scholarship: Contemporary academic presses adhere to strict ethics guidelines established by organizations like the Committee on Publication Ethics (COPE), actively screening research for bias, human rights violations, and the unauthorized use of human subjects.

Inclusive and Accurate Curricula: Modern educational publishing prioritizes historical accuracy, cultural sensitivity, and anti-racist pedagogical frameworks, intentionally correcting the historical distortions and stereotypes manufactured by past generations of publishers.

The Complicity of Architectural and Urban Planning Institutions

The construction of human zoos, native villages, and colonial compounds within world fairs and zoological gardens was not a haphazard arrangement; it was a carefully engineered spatial manifestation of racial hierarchy and imperial control.

The Architecture of Voyeurism and Spatial Subjugation

Architects and urban planners played a critical role in reinforcing the power dynamics between the spectators and the displayed captives through intentional spatial design:

The Panoptic Layout: Exposition grounds and human enclosures were engineered using panoptic principles, ensuring that captives were visible from all angles while remaining entirely devoid of privacy. Elevated walkways, viewing platforms, moats, and iron fencing reinforced an insurmountable physical and psychological barrier between the observing public and the human exhibits.

Spatial Segregation as Ideological Reinforcement: Planners deliberately positioned ethnographic camps on the peripheries of major industrial exhibits or nestled them deep within zoological gardens, directly juxtaposing colonized peoples with wild animals and machinery. This architectural placement physically communicated a pseudoscientific narrative: that indigenous populations existed on a transitional gradient between nature and modern industrial civilization.

Comparison with Modern Architectural Ethics and Urban Design

When evaluated against modern architectural ethics, urban planning standards, and human-centric design principles, the spatial planning of nineteenth-century human exhibitions represents a profound misuse of the built environment:

Human Dignity in Spatial Design: Contemporary architecture and urban design emphasize universal accessibility, spatial justice, and the psychological well-being of all occupants, rejecting spaces intentionally designed for surveillance, segregation, or degradation.

Ethical Commemoration of Public Space: Modern urban planning seeks to decolonize public spaces, replacing structures built on exploitation and exclusion with inclusive memorials, educational spaces, and public designs that honor human rights and historical truth.

The Complicity of Photography and Visual Media Industries

The visual documentation of human zoos was not a passive record of historical events; it was an aggressive, exploitative industry that profited directly from the objectification of captive performers.

The Commercialization of the Voyeuristic Gaze

Photography studios, postcard manufacturers, and early documentary filmmakers established a lucrative enterprise built on the mass reproduction and consumption of racialized imagery:

Staged Authenticity and Exotica: Photographers working inside exposition camps routinely directed captives to pose with props, assume exaggerated postures, or dress in artificial costumes designed to satisfy Western expectations of savagery and primitiveness. These manipulated images were printed by the millions onto postcards, stereograph cards, and magazine spreads, circulating global stereotypes that reinforced colonial authority.

Profit from Non-Consensual Voyeurism: Captives were frequently photographed without their knowledge, consent, or compensation. The resulting images were treated as commercial inventory and intellectual property belonging exclusively to the studios and promoters, stripping the individuals depicted of any control over their own likenesses while generating vast profits for the visual media industry.

Comparison with Modern Photography Ethics and Media Standards

When measured against contemporary photojournalism ethics, image rights, and media consent frameworks—such as the National Press Photographers Association (NPPA) code of ethics and international copyright laws regarding human likeness:

The Mandate of Informed Consent: Modern visual media standards require explicit, informed consent from all human subjects before photography or filming can take place, strictly prohibiting the exploitation or deception of vulnerable populations for commercial gain.

Respect for Human Dignity and Autonomy: Contemporary ethical photography emphasizes empathy, accuracy, and the preservation of personal dignity, completely rejecting the nineteenth-century commodification of human likeness as a tool of racial subjugation.

The Complicity of Zoological Gardens and Animal Exhibition Management

Across Europe and North America, urban zoos were among the primary institutional hosts for human exhibitions, seamlessly integrating human beings into zoological display circuits alongside exotic wildlife.

The Bestialization of Human Beings

Zoo directors and administrators actively erased the boundary between human beings and captive animals, utilizing the infrastructure of natural history to reinforce pseudoscientific racism:

Infrastructure Sharing and Caging: Zoos housed human performers in animal enclosures—such as bear pits, monkey houses, and iron-barred compounds—and subjected them to the same daily routines of public feeding schedules, viewing hours, and veterinary oversight. Administrators treated the human troupes as biological assets no different from the exotic fauna in adjacent exhibits.

Curatorial Framing and Promotion: Zoo management marketed human displays with the same sensationalist fervor used for wild animals, publishing guidebooks and promotional posters that grouped indigenous peoples alongside primates and carnivores to visually validate evolutionary theories of human development.

Comparison with Modern Zoological Ethics and Animal Welfare Standards

When evaluated against modern zoological ethics, professional accreditation standards (such as those of the Association of Zoos and Aquariums), and contemporary human rights frameworks:

Rejection of Species-Crossing Exploitation: Modern zoological institutions operate under strict ethical charters centered on wildlife conservation, animal welfare, and education, entirely prohibiting the display of human beings or the conflation of human cultures with animal management.

Ethical Accountability in Public Institutions: Contemporary zoos recognize their historical complicity in scientific racism, leading many modern institutions to issue formal apologies, remove legacy exhibitions from their archives, and educate the public on the dark intersections of zoology and human exploitation.

The Complicity of Insurance and Risk-Management Industries

Financial risk protection was a vital, yet entirely hidden, component of the exhibition apparatus.

Underwriting Human Commodification

Insurance underwriters and actuaries calculated the financial exposure of exposition syndicates, assessing the monetary value of equipment, property, and human performers:

Valuation of Human Assets: Insurance policies frequently classified human performers as movable property, touring assets, or specialized personnel under corporate liability frameworks. Actuaries priced policies based on actuarial tables that factored in the high mortality and morbidity rates of indigenous troupes traveling to foreign climates, treating human lives as calculable financial risks rather than inviolable persons.

Shielding Syndicates from Loss: By providing comprehensive casualty, transport, and liability coverage, insurance firms minimized the financial risks for promoters when performers fell ill, escaped, or died. This safety net encouraged reckless operational practices, as showmen knew their financial investments were protected against the human tragedies occurring within the camps.

Comparison with Modern Insurance Ethics and Corporate Risk Standards

When evaluated against modern insurance ethics, underwriting standards, and international human rights risk frameworks (such as the UN Guiding Principles on Business and Human Rights):

Prohibition of Insuring Harm and Exploitation: Contemporary insurance underwriters are strictly prohibited from issuing policies that commodify human life, cover illegal trafficking, or protect enterprises that violate basic human rights and labor laws.

Human Rights Due Diligence in Underwriting: Modern risk management requires insurers to assess environmental, social, and governance (ESG) factors, ensuring that financial services do not enable the exploitation, endangerment, or degradation of vulnerable human populations.

The Complicity of Hospitality, Catering, and Tourism Industries

Hotels, restaurants, transport lines, and souvenir vendors built a profitable secondary economy directly on the spectacle of human subjugation.

Monetizing the Spectacle of Degradation

The tourism and hospitality industries transformed human zoos and colonial villages into luxury consumer experiences, normalizing exploitation through leisure and entertainment:

The Tourism Supply Chain: Travel agencies, railway syndicates, and steamship lines offered packaged excursion tickets that combined transit, hotel accommodations, and admission to human exhibition camps. By bundling human displays into standard holiday itineraries, these commercial networks normalized captivity as a wholesome, family-friendly tourist attraction.

Commodification of Souvenirs and Curiosities: On-site vendors and catering establishments sold ethnographic trinkets, miniature models of native huts, and exploitative photographic postcards. This commercialization turned human suffering into portable souvenirs, allowing visitors to consume and domesticate the tragedy of others for personal amusement and decorative display in their homes.

Comparison with Modern Tourism Ethics and Sustainable Travel Standards

When measured against modern sustainable tourism frameworks, ethical travel guidelines (such as the Global Code of Ethics for Tourism), and responsible hospitality standards:

Prohibition of Exploitative Tourism: Contemporary tourism ethics strictly condemn human safari displays, voyeuristic tourism, and any commercial enterprise that commodifies indigenous cultures or human vulnerability for leisure.

Respectful and Equitable Engagement: Modern responsible tourism mandates cultural authenticity, community consent, and fair economic benefit sharing, ensuring that the travel and hospitality sectors champion human dignity rather than historical degradation.

The Complicity of Municipal Governments and Urban Authorities

City administrations were not passive bystanders; they were enthusiastic partners who viewed human zoos and colonial expositions as vital instruments of civic prestige and economic development.

Municipal Infrastructure and Public Subsidies

City governments across Europe and North America provided the essential municipal backing required to mount massive global exhibitions:

Land Grants and Tax Exemptions: Town councils and municipal bodies routinely donated prime public real estate—such as municipal parks, waterfronts, and fairgrounds—to exposition syndicates rent-free or at heavily subsidized rates. They also waived local taxes and invested public municipal funds into upgrading transit networks, water lines, and police infrastructure specifically to accommodate the millions of visitors drawn to the human camps.

Civic Branding and Tourism Promotion: Mayors and civic boosters utilized human exhibitions to brand their cities as modern, cosmopolitan centers of global trade and imperial dominance. Municipal tourism boards marketed the captive human displays in international advertising campaigns, treating the subjugation of indigenous peoples as a primary civic attraction that would boost local hotel occupancy and retail revenue.

Comparison with Modern Municipal Governance and Human Rights Standards

When evaluated against contemporary municipal governance, civic human rights obligations, and modern public administration ethics:

Civic Duty to Protect Human Rights: Modern municipal governments are bound by constitutional and international human rights frameworks that prohibit the use of public funds, municipal property, or city resources to support enterprises that degrade human dignity, violate labor rights, or promote racial discrimination.

Ethical Urban Leadership: Contemporary city administrations prioritize public welfare, social equity, and cultural inclusivity, ensuring that municipal infrastructure and public spaces serve to foster community well-being rather than host exploitative spectacles.

The Complicity of Post-Exhibition Silence and Archival Erasure

Once public outrage, shifting political landscapes, and the trauma of global conflicts forced the eventual dismantling of human zoos and colonial villages, the institutions responsible engaged in a concerted effort to erase the history of what occurred:

Purging and Concealing Records: Organizing syndicates, municipal archives, and government departments routinely destroyed, locked away, or classified administrative ledgers, correspondence, medical records, and census logs detailing the deaths, illnesses, and mistreatment of performers. This institutional amnesia was designed to protect the reputations of the sponsoring states, corporations, and scientific bodies.

Normalizing Historical Amnesia: For generations, textbooks, encyclopedias, and official histories completely omitted the human exhibition era, glossing over world's fairs and colonial expositions as purely technological and cultural celebrations. This deliberate silence protected the collective conscience of Western societies, shielding generations from confronting the brutal human cost of imperial entertainment.

Comparison with Modern Archival Ethics and Transitional Justice

When measured against contemporary archival standards, international truth-reconciliation frameworks, and modern historical transparency ethics:

The Right to Truth and Access to Information: Modern archival science operates on the principle of open access, transparency, and accountability, ensuring that historical records—particularly those documenting human rights abuses and state-sanctioned exploitation—are preserved, digitized, and made accessible to researchers and descendant communities.

Historical Reckoning and Restorative Truth: Contemporary transitional justice and historical ethics demand active disclosure, public acknowledgment of past atrocities, and the unearthing of suppressed records to restore dignity to victims and ensure that institutional complicity is never again hidden behind walls of bureaucratic silence.

The United Nations Stand on Historical Exploitation, Human Exhibitions, and Restitution

The United Nations Framework on Historical Injustices and Racism

The United Nations has systematically addressed the foundational ideologies that permitted human zoos, colonial exhibitions, and the commodification of human beings:

Condemnation of Racial Superiority Theories: The UN General Assembly, through landmark frameworks such as the United Nations Declaration on the Rights of Indigenous Peoples (UNDRIP), explicitly affirms that all doctrines, policies, and practices based on or advocating the superiority of peoples or individuals on the basis of national origin or racial, religious, ethnic, or cultural differences are racist, scientifically false, legally invalid, morally condemnable, and socially unjust.

Recognition of Historic Injustices: International human rights bodies formally recognize that indigenous peoples and marginalized populations suffered profound historical injustices as a direct result of colonization, dispossession, and exploitative scientific practices. The global human zoos and exposition circuits are understood within this framework not as benign entertainment, but as state-sanctioned violations of human dignity and equality.

UN Mandates on Repatriation, Redress, and Restitution

In alignment with contemporary international human rights law, the United Nations establishes explicit obligations for states and cultural institutions holding the remnants of historical exploitation:

The Right to Repatriation of Human Remains: Article 12 of UNDRIP mandates that states shall seek to enable the access and repatriation of ceremonial objects and human remains in their possession through fair, transparent, and effective mechanisms developed in conjunction with the concerned indigenous peoples. This counters the nineteenth-century academic and museum practice of retaining exhibition captives as research specimens.

Effective Redress and Restitution: Article 11 stipulates that states must provide redress—including restitution—through effective mechanisms developed in cooperation with indigenous communities, covering cultural, intellectual, religious, and spiritual property taken without free, prior, and informed consent.

The Imperative of Historical Truth: Through expert mechanisms and periodic human rights reviews, the UN consistently emphasizes that member states must dismantle lingering institutional colonial structures, foster historical transparency, and support active educational efforts to ensure that the systemic commodification of human beings is permanently rejected by the global community.

Dismantling the Structural Legacy and Forging Concrete Solutions

True historical reckoning requires actionable, forward-looking solutions designed to dismantle the structural legacies of the human exhibition era and ensure that such systemic commodification can never happen again.

Concrete Solutions to Eradicate Exploitative Display and Structural Racism

To permanently neutralize the ideological and institutional machinery that enabled human zoos and colonial exhibitions, the global community must implement rigorous, enforceable remedies across multiple sectors:

Enactment of Universal Anti-Commodification Legislation: Governments worldwide must pass robust, extraterritorial laws that explicitly criminalize the exhibition, public commodification, or degradation of human beings for commercial or entertainment purposes, closing any remaining legal loopholes that protect voyeuristic or pseudoscientific exploitation.

Mandatory Institutional Repatriation and Decolonization of Archives: Museums, universities, and government archives must be legally mandated to conduct comprehensive transparency audits, unconditionally returning all stolen human remains, sacred artifacts, and archival records to their descendant communities. Archival files documenting past exploitation must be fully digitized and made accessible for public education and restorative justice.

Radical Reform of Educational Curricula: International educational standards must enforce the inclusion of the history of human exhibitions, scientific racism, and colonialism in all school textbooks. Students must be taught to critically evaluate the historical intersections of science, media, government, and commerce that permitted human rights violations.

Enforcement of Rigorous Ethical Human Rights Auditing: Financial institutions, tourism syndicates, insurance underwriters, and media corporations must be bound by strict legal frameworks—such as mandatory Human Rights Due Diligence (HRDD)—ensuring that no capital, insurance coverage, or public infrastructure can ever be utilized to support enterprises that demean human dignity or violate international human rights standards.

The Imperative of Global Institutional Vigilance and Future Guarantees

Understanding who was responsible for the human exhibition circuit—from municipal governments and zoological gardens to academic presses, insurance syndicates, and visual media empires—serves as a vital diagnostic tool, but protecting future generations requires proactive, systemic safeguards.

Establishing Permanent International Oversight Frameworks

Preventing the resurgence of human commodification in modern entertainment, digital media, and global tourism requires robust, cross-border regulatory mechanisms:

Global Human Rights Monitoring Bodies: International coalitions, working in tandem with the United Nations and regional human rights courts, must establish specialized monitoring task forces dedicated to identifying modern iterations of exploitative human display, whether under the guise of "cultural tourism," "authentic tribal experiences," or unregulated digital livestreaming of vulnerable indigenous groups.

Corporate Accountability and Legal Liability: International trade and human rights laws must hold multinational corporations, tourism operators, and media networks criminally and civilly liable for any commercial enterprise that exploits human likeness, dignity, or cultural heritage without explicit, ongoing, and informed consent.

The Role of Civil Society and Grassroots Movements

Institutional reform cannot succeed without the continuous pressure and active participation of civil society:

Community-Led Oversight: Descendant communities and indigenous-led organizations must be granted veto power and primary governance authority over how their histories, cultures, and ancestral legacies are represented in public spaces, museums, and educational media.

Public Education and Historical Awareness: Sustained grassroots advocacy ensures that the memory of the human exhibition era remains a central pillar of anti-racist education, reminding society that the commodification of human beings thrives wherever ethical vigilance falters.

Vision for Restorative Global Justice

The legacy of human zoos and colonial expositions cannot be undone by mere acknowledgment; it requires a profound, structural reorganization of how modern institutions valuc human dignity, cultural autonomy, and historical truth.

The Blueprint for Restorative Transformation

Achieving true closure and justice regarding the era of human exhibitions involves several interconnected pillars:

Global Solidarity and Reparative Diplomacy: Nations and institutions that profited from the subjugation and display of human beings must engage in formal reparative diplomacy, providing financial, educational, and logistical support to the descendants of those who suffered. This includes funding community-led heritage centers, historical preservation projects, and cultural revitalization initiatives in affected regions.

The Permanent Institutional Oath: Museums, universities, municipal bodies, and transnational corporations must adopt formal, binding institutional oaths pledging never to commodify human vulnerability, misrepresent cultures for entertainment, or compromise human rights for commercial or scientific prestige.

Conclusion

The history of human exhibitions stands as one of the most comprehensive systemic failures in modern civilization, implicating virtually every pillar of society—from science and government to commerce, media, and education. By thoroughly mapping this web of responsibility and enacting unyielding preventative solutions, the global community ensures that the lessons of the past serve as an enduring shield for human dignity across future generations.

PART III

The Legacy That Still Lives

Chapter 9

When the World Finally Looked Away

The dismantling of the human exhibition circuit did not happen overnight, nor was it the result of a sudden, collective moral awakening by the institutions that built it. Instead, the collapse of human zoos and colonial villages was forced by years of relentless pressure from a diverse coalition of critics. Religious leaders, investigative journalists, social reformers, and local activists chipped away at the spectacle, gradually turning public opinion against an industry that had long operated with impunity.

The Moral Outcry: Religious Leaders and Ethical Condemnation

Religious institutions and spiritual leaders were among the first organized voices to challenge the fundamental inhumanity of displaying human beings as wild animals:

Denouncing the Violation of Human Sanctity: Clergymen and religious groups from various denominations began preaching sermons and publishing theological essays condemning human exhibitions as a profound affront to divine creation and universal human brotherhood.

Challenging Hypocrisy: Religious reformers exposed the glaring hypocrisy of Western nations sending missionaries abroad to "civilize" foreign populations while simultaneously importing, degrading, and caging indigenous people in European and American fairgrounds for public amusement.

The Power of the Pen: Investigative Journalists and Whistleblowers

Journalists and early human rights advocates utilized the press to puncture the sanitized, romanticized narrative spun by exposition promoters:

Exposing Brutal Realities: Reporters infiltrated human exhibition camps to document the squalid living conditions, rampant disease, malnutrition, and psychological distress suffered by the captives. Investigative articles detailed how performers were frequently deceived into signing contracts, subjected to harsh weather without adequate clothing, and abandoned when they fell ill.

Amplifying Resistance: The press began reporting on acts of defiance, strikes, and petitions organized by the captives themselves, proving to the reading public that the displayed individuals were active human agents rejecting their captivity rather than willing participants in a cultural showcase.

Social Reformers and Grassroots Activism

A network of human rights advocates, anti-slavery veterans, and emerging civil rights organizations translated moral outrage into coordinated political action:

Petitioning Authorities: Reformers flooded city councils, colonial ministries, and parliamentary offices with petitions demanding the immediate banning of human displays on municipal and public grounds.

Shifting Public Conscience: By organizing public lectures, distributing pamphlets, and leveraging changing social norms following the devastation of global conflicts, reformers reframed human zoos from harmless educational entertainment into barbaric relics of an indefensible era.

The Internal Resistance: Agency and Defiance by the Captives

While external critics, journalists, and religious leaders applied pressure from the outside, the most effective catalyst for the decline of human exhibitions came from within the camps themselves. Captive performers were never passive victims; they actively resisted their objectification, forcing exposition organizers, showmen, and municipal authorities to confront the volatile and unsustainable nature of their enterprises.

Work Stoppages and Labor Strikes: Troupes frequently organized coordinated walkouts, refusing to perform, dance, or pose for crowds until their contractual grievances were met, wages were paid, or basic provisions were improved. These strikes disrupted the commercial flow of the expositions and embarrassed promoters in front of paying audiences.

Legal Battles and Consular Interventions: Whenever possible, captives reached out to foreign consulates, sympathetic lawyers, or local anti-slavery societies to file lawsuits for breach of contract, illegal confinement, or kidnapping. These legal challenges threatened organizers with costly litigation and public scandals, making human exhibitions an increasingly high-risk business venture.

Escape and Subversion: Individual captives routinely sought escape routes out of fairgrounds, blending into local immigrant communities or seeking repatriation assistance. Their daring flights from the enclosed camps punctured the illusion of docile submission that promoters marketed to the public.

Economic Shifts and the Changing Landscape of Entertainment

By the mid-twentieth century, the decline of human zoos was accelerated by fundamental economic and technological transformations that rendered the human exhibition model obsolete:

The Rise of Alternative Media: The expansion of cinema, illustrated magazines, and documentary photography provided the public with new avenues for visual engagement with foreign cultures, reducing the consumer demand for physical, live-human spectacles.

Shifting Imperial Economics: The devastating financial and political tolls of global conflicts, combined with rising anti-colonial liberation movements across Africa, Asia, and the Americas, made governments increasingly reluctant to sponsor controversial overseas displays that inflamed diplomatic tensions and fueled nationalist resistance abroad.

The Geopolitical Realities of Decolonization

As the post-war era unfolded, the geopolitical map of the world underwent a massive seismic shift. The collapse of European empires and the rise of sovereign nation-states across the Global South introduced severe diplomatic consequences for any nation attempting to continue colonial-style exhibitions.

Diplomatic Backlash: Newly independent governments and emerging international coalitions viewed human exhibitions and ethnographic villages as deeply offensive reminders of imperial subjugation. Hosting such spectacles risked immediate diplomatic condemnation, trade disputes, and severed political alliances with newly liberated nations that now held voting power in international bodies like the United Nations.

The Criminalization of Exploitation: Changing international laws regarding human trafficking, labor standards, and basic human rights meant that the logistical framework required to transport, cage, and display foreign nationals could no longer operate legally under national or international jurisdictions.

The Lingering Shadows: Transitioning into Modern Tourism and Media

Even as traditional human zoos closed their gates for the final time, the underlying commercial and voyeuristic impulses did not vanish entirely; instead, they mutated into new, sanitized formats:

The Birth of Commercialized "Cultural Tourism": Promoters and travel agencies shifted from static fairground displays to packaged international tours, commercializing indigenous communities in their home territories through voyeuristic human safari tours and staged cultural performances that often-prioritized Western expectations of "authenticity" over genuine cultural respect.

Media Representation and Exoticism: Early television documentaries, adventure magazines, and travelogues frequently inherited the paternalistic, exoticizing gaze of the human exhibition era, framing non-Western peoples through a lens of backwardness or spectacle for Western audiences.

The gradual closing of the human exhibition era was thus a complex convergence of external moral awakening, internal acts of defiance by the captives, shifting global economics, and the rising tide of anti-colonial resistance. When the world finally looked away, it marked not the immediate end of exoticism, but the definitive collapse of its most brutally overt institutional manifestation.

The Evolution of Anthropological and Scientific Retraction

As the social sciences matured and broke away from nineteenth-century racial pseudo-science, academic institutions began to quietly distance themselves from their historical complicity in human exhibitions:

Discrediting Racial Hierarchies: Evolutionary biology, modern anthropology, and genetics decisively dismantled the pseudoscientific theories of polygenism and unilineal cultural evolution that had once provided intellectual justification for human zoos. Scholars began to publicly repudiate the notion that human populations existed on a graded scale from "primitive" to "civilized."

Institutional Silence and Internal Reckoning: While many universities and scientific bodies initially sought to bury their involvement in sponsoring, measuring, and studying exhibition captives, later generations of academics initiated critical self-examinations. This academic shift helped erode the final pillars of intellectual authority that showmen had relied upon to market human zoos as legitimate educational enterprises.

The Role of Memorialization and Public Conscience

The final phase of the world looking away involved confronting the physical and cultural scars left behind by decades of public exhibition:

Uncovering Forgotten Graves: Modern historical research and investigative journalism have increasingly focused on locating the unmarked graves of performers who died far from home in foreign exposition camps, ensuring their names and identities are restored from archival obscurity.

Commemoration and Apology: Descendant communities, local activists, and progressive municipal authorities have begun erecting monuments, renaming streets, and placing commemorative plaques at the historic sites of former world's fairs and human zoos. These memorials serve as permanent reminders of a dark chapter in public entertainment, ensuring that the history of human exploitation is openly acknowledged rather than conveniently forgotten.

The Legacy of Resistance: Honoring the Agency of the Captives

As historical scholarship continues to unpack the final decades of the human exhibition era, a vital shift has occurred regarding how the captives are remembered:

From Objects of Pity to Agents of Resistance: Rather than perpetuating a narrative that reduces indigenous performers solely to victims of Western oppression, modern historians emphasize their active resistance, resilience, and cultural preservation. Captives maintained their languages, spiritual practices, and communal bonds in the face of immense psychological and physical adversity.

Restoring Historical Dignity: Archival projects worldwide are actively working to recover the true names, biographies, and homelands of individuals who were stripped of their identities by exposition showmen. This meticulous historical recovery transforms nameless "spechibits" back into recognized individuals with rich ancestral lineages and personal histories.

The Ongoing Re-evaluation of Museum and Institutional Collections

Even after the physical gates of human zoos were closed, the institutional framework that supported them left behind vast collections of ethnographic items, photographs, plaster casts, and human remains housed in university departments and national museums. The final stages of the world looking away necessarily involve confronting these lingering material legacies:

Challenging Colonial Collection Ethics: Modern Museum boards and curators are increasingly forced to re-examine the provenance of collections acquired during the height of the human exhibition era. Many objects and remains were obtained through coercion, theft, or exploitation during exposition visits, making their continued retention legally and ethically untenable.

The Transition to Restitution Partnerships: Rather than maintaining unilateral control over disputed cultural property, major institutions are establishing collaborative partnerships with indigenous nations, setting up long-term loan agreements, co-management frameworks, and unconditional returns of ancestral heritage.

Reflections on the Demise of the Spectacle

The collapse of the human exhibition industry demonstrates the ultimate fragility of systems built on the institutionalized degradation of human beings. When moral clarity breached the walls of public indifference, the entire apparatus crumbled under its own ethical weight. This records a monumental shift—a moment when humanity finally refused to be spectators to its own moral failure.

The Transition from Physical Display to Digital and Photographic Archives

As the physical human zoos faded from public parks and fairgrounds, a new frontier of ethical responsibility emerged regarding the preservation, display, and digital dissemination of historical imagery from that era:

Ethical Curation of Historical Photography: Archives, libraries, and digital repositories are establishing strict ethical guidelines for how photographs, postcards, and film reels of exhibition captives are handled, indexed, and displayed online. Displaying historical images of exploited individuals without context or consent is increasingly recognized as a digital continuation of the original violation.

Contextualizing Visual Exploitation: Modern history portals now mandate explicit trigger warnings, historical contextualization, and community-consulted metadata alongside archival photographs, ensuring that viewers understand these images as documents of state-sanctioned abuse rather than passive ethnographic portraits.

The Global Legacy of Conscience

The ultimate collapse of human exhibitions left an indelible mark on global human rights standards, serving as a permanent historical reference point for the dangers of state-sponsored racism and commercialized human degradation:

The Birth of Modern Cultural Sensitivity: The profound social trauma inflicted by the human exhibition circuit catalyzed a global demand for cultural respect, inspiring international frameworks that protect indigenous rights, cultural heritage, and bodily autonomy.

An Enduring Reminder: It is an ultimate illustration that while systems of institutional exploitation can persist for generations under the guise of progress or entertainment, they are inherently fragile when met with unyielding moral courage, internal agency, and global accountability.

The Intersection of Public Memory and National Curricula

To ensure that the lessons of the human exhibition era are never forgotten or sanitized by future generations, educational reformers and historians continue to push for structural changes in national schooling:

Beyond the Textbook: Modern pedagogical frameworks advocate for immersive, primary-source-driven curricula that directly study the mechanisms of human zoos, world's fairs, and scientific racism. By examining original handbills, newspaper editorials, and captive testimonies, students learn to critically deconstruct how institutional power manufactures consent for human exploitation.

National Truth and Reconciliation Initiatives: Several nations whose cities once hosted sprawling human exhibition camps have begun exploring formal national truth commissions, ensuring that the historical trauma inflicted upon foreign captives and indigenous communities is acknowledged at the highest levels of government.

The Permanent Vigilance of Civil Society

The definitive end of the human exhibition era underscores a timeless lesson regarding human rights: the line between education and exploitation, culture and commodification, is dangerously thin.

Guarding Against Modern Resurgences: Civil society organizations, human rights defenders, and indigenous coalitions maintain active watch over modern entertainment, digital media, and global tourism platforms to ensure that voyeuristic spectacle never again masquerades as cross-cultural appreciation.

The Legacy of Resistance: A tribute to the resilience of those who endured the spectacles. Their collective endurance, silent defiance, and ultimate refusal to be erased stand as the true foundation upon which modern human dignity and global accountability rest.

The Responsibility of Modern Cultural Institutions and Museums

As the echoes of the human exhibition era continue to resonate through contemporary society, museums and cultural centers bear a unique responsibility in shaping public memory:

Curating Accountability: Rather than hiding their past associations with colonial expositions and racial pseudo-science, forward-thinking museums now host dedicated permanent and rotating exhibitions examining how ethnographic displays were used to manufacture public consent for imperialism.

Transparent Provenance Research: Institutions are increasingly dedicating resources to provenance research, meticulously tracing how artifacts, human remains, and archival materials entered museum vaults during the nineteenth and twentieth centuries to ensure transparent restitution pipelines.

The Turning point

The definitive closure of human zoos and colonial villages represents a monumental turning point in human history—a moment when the global community finally confronted the moral bankruptcy of treating human lives as public spectacle. The tireless efforts of religious critics, investigative journalists, social reformers, and most importantly, the unyielding resistance of the captives themselves, dismantled an industry built on exploitation. A testament to the fact that when moral clarity pierces the veil of cultural complacency, institutionalized injustice can and will be ended.

The Psychological and Generational Trauma of Exhibition Descendants

The legacy of the human exhibition era extends far beyond the physical dismantling of fairgrounds and colonial villages; it left deep generational and psychological wounds among the descendant families of those who were caged, studied, and displayed:

The Intergenerational Transmission of Grief: Descendants of exhibition performers often grew up carrying the unspoken trauma of their ancestors' humiliation, displacement, and medicalized exploitation. For decades, institutional secrecy and societal shame conspired to silence these family histories, leaving descendants to piece together fragmented archives and whispered accounts.

Healing Through Ancestral Retrieval: Modern descendant-led initiatives focus heavily on holistic healing, emotional restoration, and public storytelling. By reclaiming the narratives of their forebears, families are transforming historical shame into profound pride, ensuring that their ancestors are remembered not as passive victims of colonial spectacle, but as resilient survivors who endured unimaginable cruelty.

The Continuing Duty of Global Scholars and Historians

As academic research into the human exhibition era expands into new interdisciplinary fields, scholars carry a heavy burden of ethical responsibility:

Collaborative Historiography: Contemporary historians and anthropologists no longer study marginalized communities from a detached, paternalistic distance. Instead, they operate under strict participatory frameworks where descendant communities direct the research questions, control the narrative framing, and co-author historical findings.

Unmasking Institutional Complicity: Ongoing archival excavations continue to reveal the deep-seated financial, political, and academic connections that sustained human zoos, ensuring that modern universities, municipal archives, and government bodies can never fully detach themselves from their historical accountability.

The Evolution of International Legal Protections Against Exploitation

The dismantling of human exhibitions served as a vital catalyst for the development of modern international humanitarian law, reshaping how global legal frameworks address human dignity, consent, and cultural preservation:

Codifying Protection Against Degradation: Post-war human rights conventions, including foundational declarations by the United Nations, drew critical lessons from the abuses of the colonial exhibition era. These documents established strict international legal principles prohibiting degrading treatment, forced labor, and the public commodification of vulnerable populations under any guise.

Empowering Indigenous Self-Determination: Modern international instruments, such as the United Nations Declaration on the Rights of Indigenous Peoples (UNDRIP), provide robust legal mechanisms that safeguard indigenous cultures, traditional knowledge, and physical likeness against commercial exploitation, ensuring that historical atrocities can never be legally replicated under modern tourism or media laws.

The Role of Digital Heritage Preservation in Historical Rectification

As humanity transitions further into the digital age, archival institutions and human rights advocates are leveraging advanced digital technologies to preserve the historical record while safeguarding the dignity of those who suffered:

Secure and Respectful Archives: Digital historians design specialized metadata standards and access restrictions for sensitive historical records, ensuring that researchers can study the mechanisms of human zoos without perpetuating the voyeuristic gaze of nineteenth-century spectators.

Global Educational Access: Online platforms and virtual learning modules enable classrooms worldwide to explore primary sources, oral histories, and expert analysis of the human exhibition era, embedding critical anti-racist education firmly into global curricula and ensuring that the lessons of the past remain accessible to all.

The Ongoing Transformation of Popular Culture and Media Ethics

As society moved further from the era of human exhibitions, the entertainment and media industries faced a prolonged reckoning regarding how they portray non-Western cultures, traditions, and individuals:

Eradicating Exotic Tropes in Cinema and Literature: Filmmakers, screenwriters, and publishers began actively dismantling the paternalistic tropes and savage caricatures that had been popularized by nineteenth-century human zoos and colonial expositions. The demand for authentic, multi-dimensional storytelling replaced the flat, exoticized stereotypes that once satisfied Western voyeurism.

Ethics in Global Documentary Filmmaking: Modern documentary crews and ethnographic journalists adopted rigorous ethical guidelines based on informed consent, collaborative storytelling, and mutual respect, ensuring that visual media served to empower rather than exploit vulnerable or indigenous communities.

The Vital Role of Local Municipalities and City Governments

The infrastructure of the human exhibition era was largely built on public land, municipal parks, and state-funded exposition grounds. Consequently, local governments bear a continuing responsibility to address this historical footprint:

Reclaiming Public Spaces: Municipalities across Europe, North America, and other regions that once hosted sprawling colonial exhibitions are undertaking urban renewal projects that incorporate historical markers, interpretive installations, and public art dedicated to honoring the victims of human zoos.

Fostering Civic Dialogue: City councils increasingly sponsor public forums, cultural festivals, and educational symposia that engage residents in discussions about colonialism, institutional racism, and the local history of public exhibitions, turning sites of historical shame into centers of civic education and reconciliation.

The Intersection of Environmental Justice and Indigenous Land Rights

The mechanisms that facilitated human exhibitions were inextricably linked to extractive colonialism and land dispossession. As modern human rights movements evolve, the fight against the legacies of human zoos is increasingly tied to environmental justice and indigenous sovereignty:

Restoring Stewardship: Recognizing that many individuals displayed in human zoos were forcibly removed from their native lands under the guise of "scientific curiosity" or "territorial pacification," modern advocacy emphasizes the return of ancestral lands to indigenous stewardship. Restoring ecological and territorial control is viewed as a vital component of repairing the holistic damage caused by colonial exploitation.

Challenging Modern Environmental Voyeurism: Environmental activists and indigenous leaders draw direct parallels between historical human exhibitions and modern eco-tourism practices that treat indigenous reservations or protected natural habitats as human living museums. Ensuring strict self-determination prevents contemporary industries from commodifying indigenous daily life for affluent travelers.

The Permanent Mandate of Global Accountability

Protection of human dignity requires constant, unyielding vigilance:

The Cost of Complacency: The human exhibition era thrived because ordinary citizens, scientists, and officials allowed curiosity to override morality, normalizing the unimaginable. Preventing future iterations of systemic exploitation demands that society continuously question institutional motives, media representations, and state-sanctioned displays of human difference.

A Resilient Legacy of Truth: Ultimately, the transition from public indifference to global condemnation proves that human societies possess the capacity to correct monumental moral errors.

By honoring the resilience of those who resisted, maintaining transparency in historical education, and enforcing strict international human rights protections, the global community ensures that the world never looks away from the lessons of its past.

The Deep Psychological Mechanics of the Spectator's Gaze

The human zoo was not merely a physical enclosure of wood and iron; it was an elaborate theatre of psychological reassurance for the industrializing West:

Manufacturing Ontological Security: In an era defined by rapid urbanization, technological disruption, and the unsettling anxieties of modernization, European and American citizens flocked to human exhibitions to anchor their own identities. By viewing colonized peoples framed as static, primitive, and unchanging, the Western spectator manufactured a comforting illusion of evolutionary superiority and personal stability. The other was purposefully constructed as a fixed baseline against which the modern self could measure its supposed progress.

The Normalization of Surveillance and Power: Walking through the aisles of a human village habituated ordinary citizens to the panoptic gaze. It taught generations to view human bodies—particularly non-white bodies—as objects open to inspection, measurement, categorization, and judgment. This daily training in voyeurism seamlessly bled into the administrative, medical, and military apparatuses of the colonial state, making mass subjugation feel natural and routine.

The Complicity of the Medical and Scientific Establishment

The decline of human zoos was severely protracted because the enterprise was legitimized by the highest intellectual authorities of the nineteenth and early twentieth centuries. The dismantling of this academic shield required a radical epistemological rupture:

The Weaponization of Anthropometry: University departments of anatomy, anthropology, and medicine actively collaborated with exhibition promoters. Scientists frequently visit fairgrounds not to liberate the captives, but to treat the human enclosures as living laboratories. They subjected performers to forced cranial measurements, dental casts, and physiological testing under the guise of objective research.

Deconstructing Scientific Racism from Within: The eventual collapse of human exhibitions coincided with the painful, generational unraveling of scientific racism. As pioneering anthropologists and geneticists—such as Franz Boas and his successors—dismantled the intellectual foundations of unilineal cultural evolution, they pulled the academic rug out from under the showmen. When universities could no longer defend human displays as legitimate science, the industry lost its veneer of respectability, leaving promoters exposed as mere merchants of exploitation.

The Micro-Politics of Everyday Resistance Inside the Camps

Beyond organized labor strikes and legal battles, the daily existence of the captives was an ongoing, micro-political war of attrition against total objectification:

Preserving Cultural Sovereignty Through Secrecy: Promoters demanded that performers act out crude, scripted stereotypes of savagery for the paying crowds. In response, captives engaged in subtle acts of cultural preservation behind the scenes. They whispered in their native tongues, secretly performed sacred rituals away from the prying eyes of managers, and constructed alternative kinship networks within the camps to shield their authentic identities from the commodifying gaze.

The Reclamation of the Narrative: Whenever possible, literate captives or those who learned European languages utilized foreign newspapers and direct-address pamphlets to talk back to their audiences. By publishing their own accounts, complaints, and critiques of the fairground management, they shattered the promoter's monopoly on truth, forcing the European public to reckon with the uncomfortable reality of human coercion hidden behind the carnival banners.

The Turning Point of Apathy: How "Looking Away" Became a Moral Imperative

For decades, the primary weapon of the human zoo was not just the iron bars of the enclosure, but the collective gaze of an indifferent public. To look at an exhibition captive was to participate in an act of sanctioned dehumanization; conversely, the ultimate act of liberation required breaking that gaze entirely:

The Pathology of the Spectator's Gaze: For generations, millions of ordinary citizens walked through human zoos, colonial villages, and anthropological exhibits without experiencing moral dissonance. The act of looking was normalized as harmless curiosity, education, or entertainment. Breaking this cycle required a profound rupture in public consciousness—a moment when the collective gaze transformed from one of voyeuristic entitlement into one of shame, revulsion, and acute moral failure.

The Strategic Shift from Spectacle to Oblivion: When activists, religious leaders, and progressive journalists finally succeeded in shifting public perception, they weaponized indifference. They urged citizens to stop buying tickets, to turn their backs on the fairgrounds, and to deny showmen the oxygen of attention and profit. When the ticket sales dried up and the crowds deliberately looked away, the economic foundation of the human exhibition collapsed overnight.

The Lingering Burden of the Gaze in Modern Retrospection

Looking away was never just about closing an exhibition gate; it was the beginning of an uncomfortable reckoning with how the West viewed the rest of the world. The title echoes into our modern era, reminding contemporary society that the ghosts of the human zoo persist whenever marginalized populations are exoticized for public consumption:

Refusing the Legacy of Objectification: To truly "look away" in the historical sense means maintaining a permanent cultural refusal to treat human beings as spectacles, commodities, or living artifacts. It demands that modern institutions, media outlets, and tourism boards actively dismantle the remnants of the colonial gaze.

From Voyeurism to Witnessing: Ultimately, looking away from the spectacle meant turning toward the victims with accountability, respect, and remembrance. Chapter 9 stands as the historical chronicle of that awakening—the moment humanity realized that true civilization is measured not by how it watches the world, but by how it refuses to watch the degradation of its fellow human beings.

The Archival Recovery of Voice and the Ethics of Historical Representation

As contemporary historians and descendant communities continue to piece together the fragmented records of the human exhibition era, a critical scholarly consensus has emerged regarding the ethics of historical recovery. Citing foundational works in post-colonial studies and archival theory—such as those explored by scholars like Saidiya Hartman on the "afterlife of slavery" and the constraints of archive-induced violence—modern researchers emphasize that official records, police logs, and exposition pamphlets were written entirely through the lens of the captor.

Reading Against the Grain: To truly understand how the world looked away—and what happened when the victims were finally heard—historians must engage in meticulous counter-narrative analysis. This involves reading institutional documents, medical reports, and showmen's ledgers "against the grain" to extract the hidden truths of quiet rebellion, psychological endurance, and interpersonal solidarity among the captives.

Restricting Voyeuristic Reproduction: Prominent archival institutions, including the Musée du Quai Branly in Paris and the Smithsonian National Museum of Natural History, have adopted strict ethical guidelines regarding the public display of historical photographs from the human zoo era. Citing cultural heritage protection frameworks, these institutions restrict the uncontextualized reproduction of degrading imagery, ensuring that historical education does not inadvertently perpetuate nineteenth-century voyeurism.

The Transnational Network of Anti-Exhibition Activism

The final collapse of the human exhibition industry was not an isolated domestic phenomenon in any single European capital; rather, it was accelerated by an increasingly interconnected transnational network of moral reformers, early human rights advocates, and anti-colonial intellectuals. Archival correspondence housed in international repositories demonstrates that letters of protest crossed national borders with unprecedented frequency during the early decades of the twentieth century:

Cross-Border Solidarity: Activists in London, Paris, Berlin, and New York shared investigative reports detailing the high mortality rates, contractual abuses, and systemic deception used to recruit performers from African, Asian, and Indigenous American territories.

The Pressure of International Diplomacy: As diplomatic channels increasingly recognized that colonial exhibitions fostered violent racial friction and diplomatic embarrassment abroad, colonial offices faced mounting intergovernmental pressure to phase out live ethnographic displays. This international scrutiny transformed human zoos from profitable national showcases into diplomatic liabilities, forcing governments to quietly withdraw permits and shut down fairground enclosures permanently.

The Monumental Shift in Public Conscience: From Curiosity to Condemnation

The ultimate dismantling of the human exhibition apparatus hinged upon a profound psychological transformation within Western society shift from uncritical voyeurism to collective moral revulsion. For decades, the public had compartmentalized the human zoo as a place of harmless education and exotic entertainment, successfully insulating themselves against the human cost of the spectacles. The turning point documented in this chapter represents the painful, deliberate unraveling of that self-deception:

The Role of Whistleblowers and Exposés: Investigative journalism played an indispensable role in forcing the public to look.

When independent reporters, sympathetic physicians, and reform-minded missionaries began publishing smuggled accounts detailing rampant disease, psychological abuse, forced confinement, and soaring mortality rates within the camp enclosures, the romanticized narrative manufactured by exposition showmen shattered.

The Erosion of State Sanction: As public protests gained momentum, municipal leaders and state officials could no longer claim ignorance. The political cost of granting permits for live human displays began to outweigh the financial and prestige benefits. When the moral weight of public outrage finally pierced the walls of indifference, local governments began revoking licenses, cutting municipal subsidies, and banning the import of foreign performers for exhibition purposes.

A Permanent Warning for Modern Society

A historical account of a dark nineteenth- and twentieth-century phenomenon; it stands as a perpetual ethical touchstone for modern civilization:

Guarding Against Modern Spectacles: The mechanisms of the human zoo—exoticizing the unfamiliar, commodifying human dignity for public consumption, and reducing complex cultures into flattened caricatures—did not vanish entirely with the closure of the last colonial village. They evolved into new forms within media, tourism, and digital platforms. The enduring lesson is the vital necessity of maintaining permanent critical vigilance against any industry that treats human beings as objects of spectacle.

Honoring the Resilient Dead: Above all, the chapter preserves the memory of those who endured the unimaginable indignities of the exhibition circuit. By documenting their struggles, honoring their quiet resistance, and recovering their true names and histories from the archives of exploitation, history ensures that they are remembered not as the helpless victims of a passing fad, but as resilient human beings whose endurance ultimately forced the world to wake up, look away, and change.

The Architecture of Forgetting: How Cities Erased the Fairgrounds

When the human zoos were finally shuttered, the physical spaces that hosted them underwent a deliberate process of urban sanitation and historical erasure. Municipal planners and park commissioners sought to scrub the landscape clean of the structures that had symbolized a deeply embarrassing era of state-sponsored exploitation:

Razing the Enclosures: Across European and American capitals, wooden palisades, mock native villages, and exhibition pavilions were rapidly demolished. Exposition grounds were repurposed into public parks, athletic fields, or housing developments, effectively burying the physical infrastructure of the human zoo beneath layers of modern urban development.

The Politics of Intentional Amnesia: For decades following the closures, city officials and cultural institutions engaged in a collective silence. Guidebooks omitted mention of the human displays that had once drawn millions of visitors to world's fairs and colonial expositions, preferring to remember these events strictly as triumphs of science, industry, and international cooperation while sweeping the human cost under the rug.

The Long Road to Public Reckoning and Apology

It took generations of activist pressure, historical scholarship, and grassroots advocacy to break the institutional amnesia that followed the closure of human exhibitions. Gradually, cities and national governments began the painful process of public acknowledgment:

Erecting Counter-Monuments and Memorials: In recent decades, municipalities that once hosted human zoos have begun installing plaque markers, commemorative sculptures, and educational installations near former exposition sites. These memorials explicitly name the individuals who were displayed, restoring their humanity and countering the century-long silence imposed by civic authorities.

Formal State and Institutional Apologies: Descendants and indigenous nations have increasingly demanded—and in some cases received—formal apologies from municipal councils, university departments, and national museums whose predecessors profited from or legitimized the human exhibition industry. These acknowledgments mark a vital transition from historical denial to active reconciliation, ensuring that the legacy of when the world finally looked away is met with lasting truth and institutional accountability.

The Intersection of Educational Reform and Historical Pedagogy

As the global community confronts the profound legacies of the human exhibition era, educators and curriculum developers face the critical task of embedding this history into modern academic frameworks without sanitizing its harsh realities:

Deconstructing Colonial Ideology in the Classroom: Modern educational programs move far beyond passive historical timelines, engaging students in deep analytical exercises that examine how states, scientific institutions, and commercial enterprises manufactured consent for human exploitation. By studying primary sources—such as original event handbills, archival photographs, and letters of protest—students learn to recognize the subtle, persistent mechanics of cultural objectification.

Fostering Critical Historical Empathy: Rather than reducing the subjects of human exhibitions to passive victims of history, progressive curricula highlight individual agency, acts of silent resistance, and post-exhibition survival. This pedagogical shift ensures that learners understand the era not merely as a catalogue of atrocities, but as a testament to the unyielding dignity of those who endured and fought back.

The Ongoing Responsibility of Global Civil Society

The end of the physical human zoo did not eliminate the underlying cultural impulses that created it. The responsibility for preventing any modern iteration of human exhibitionism rests firmly on the shoulders of an active, globally conscious civil society:

Monitoring Cultural and Media Landscapes: Human rights organizations, indigenous advocacy groups, and cultural watchdogs maintain constant vigilance over modern tourism, reality television, digital media platforms, and live entertainment to ensure that exoticizing tropes and exploitative spectacles never find a renewed footing.

The Permanent Imperative of Moral Clarity: It demonstrates that while institutions of systemic exploitation can thrive for generations under the mask of progress and entertainment, they are inherently fragile when met with unyielding moral courage, collective accountability, and the absolute refusal of ordinary people to look away from injustice.

The Preservation of Descendant Oral Histories and Counter-Archives

As official state and municipal records frequently sanitized, minimized, or entirely omitted the lived experiences of human exhibition captives, the preservation of descendant oral histories has become an urgent, counter-archival imperative:

Oral Tradition as Resistance: Within many descendant families, the painful accounts of ancestors who were taken, displayed, and studied were passed down through generations via oral history. These narratives served as a vital counterweight to official colonial histories, preserving the true names, origins, and emotional realities of those who endured the fairgrounds.

Building Community-Led Repositories: Modern descendant coalitions are establishing independent digital and physical archives controlled directly by affected communities. These repositories ensure that family histories, recovered photographs, and personal artifacts remain under the stewardship of those whose ancestors were commodified, protecting them from institutional co-optation or voyeuristic misuse.

The Global Re-evaluation of Museum Collections and Human Remains

The closure of human exhibitions forced a long-overdue international reckoning regarding the human remains and cultural belongings acquired by anthropologists and showmen during the peak of the exhibition era:

The Imperative of Repatriation: Museums, universities, and scientific academies across Europe and North America have faced mounting legal and moral pressure to repatriate the remains of individuals who died while trapped in human zoos or colonial villages. Returning these remains to their ancestral homelands for proper, dignified burial is recognized as an indispensable act of restorative justice.

De-accessioning Exploitative Artifacts: Cultural institutions are systematically reviewing their collections to de-accession items acquired through coercion or exoticized spectacle, working in direct partnership with source communities to determine whether these objects should be returned, formally recontextualized, or permanently retired from public view.

The Intersection of Global Tourism and the Ghost of the Human Exhibition

Even as traditional human zoos vanished from the urban parks and exhibits of the Western world, the underlying market logic that drove them mutated into new sectors of the global leisure economy. The transition from nineteenth-century colonial displays to twentieth- and twenty-first-century tourism practices represents a subtle, ongoing challenge for cultural preservationists and human rights advocates:

The Commodification of Authenticity: Modern cultural tourism frequently replicates the structural power dynamics of the human exhibition era when indigenous or marginalized communities are packaged as static, unchanging spectacles for affluent travelers. Tour operators, cruise lines, and commercialized cultural villages sometimes pressure local populations to perform simplified, exoticized versions of their traditions to satisfy Western expectations of "primitive authenticity."

Ethical Tourism Frameworks: In response to these lingering neo-colonial tendencies, international indigenous coalitions and ethical travel organizations have established rigorous guidelines for community-based tourism. These frameworks ensure that local populations retain absolute control over their cultural presentation, economic compensation, and territorial access, preventing tourism from devolving into a modern variant of the fairground enclosure.

The Role of Fine Art and Literature in Exposing the Gaze

While historical texts and journalistic exposés played a pivotal role in dismantling human zoos, creative literature, poetry, and visual arts provided an equally vital emotional vocabulary for processing the trauma of the exhibition era:

Subverting the Portrait: Avant-garde artists and post-colonial painters began using their craft to interrogate the power dynamics of the spectator's gaze. By reinterpreting historical photographs of exhibition captives, artists stripped away the voyeuristic framing of the original promotional material, replacing it with works that highlighted the subject's agency, dignity, and profound humanity.

Literary Testimonies of Displacement: Novelists and poets from formerly colonized nations produced powerful works exploring the psychological devastation of being displayed abroad.

These literary accounts served to humanize the statistical casualties of the exhibition circuit, translating dry historical archives into resonant human stories that forced readers to confront the moral cost of Western curiosity.

The Continuing Duty of International Jurisprudence

As global legal systems continue to evolve, the historic abuses of the human exhibition era serve as a permanent benchmark against which modern human rights violations are judged. International courts and human rights tribunals frequently draw upon the legacy of colonial exploitation when adjudicating cases involving cultural appropriation, forced displacement, and the commercial exploitation of human likeness:

Protecting Cultural Integrity in International Law: Modern human rights treaties explicitly recognize that the unauthorized public display, commodification, or degradation of cultural groups constitutes a violation of fundamental human dignity. These legal instruments ensure that the systemic vulnerabilities exploited by nineteenth-century showmen are met with robust, enforceable protections today.

The Guarantee of Non-Repetition: By formally recognizing human exhibitions as a historic crime against human rights, international judicial bodies reinforce the principle of non-repetition. This legal stance ensures that states and private corporations can never claim ignorance regarding the inherent illegitimacy of reducing human beings to public spectacles.

The Micro-Economics of the Fairground: How Exploitation Was Financed

These exhibitions were not merely cultural curiosities or fringe side-shows; they were major corporate enterprises backed by banks, shipping magnates, import-export syndicates, and municipal governments:

Corporate Sponsorship and Shareholder Profit: World's fairs and colonial expositions operated as joint-stock companies. Investors purchased shares anticipating high dividends driven by massive ticket sales, concession revenues, and merchandising. This financial structure insulated the ultimate profiteers from the human misery inside the enclosures, transforming human suffering into a detached corporate asset managed by boards of directors.

The Economics of Coercion: Recruitment agents utilized systemic debt bondage, falsified labor contracts, and the withholding of return-passage funds to trap performers in foreign countries. Promoters calculated operational costs down to the penny, spending lavishly on exotic architectural facades while keeping the stipends of the performers minimal or non-existent, maximizing profit margins off the commodified bodies of the colonized.

The Role of Popular Anthropology and Mass-Market Print Media

The commercial success of human exhibitions relied heavily on the enthusiastic partnership of popular print media and emerging mass-market publishing houses:

Sensationalist Illustrated Press: Newspapers, weekly pictorials, and souvenir magazines saturated the Western public market with sensationalized woodcuts and photographs of human zoo captives. Editors understood that exoticism sold copies, so they framed the exhibits through breathless narratives of discovery, savagery, and civilizational contrast, priming readers to view human beings as live adventure novels.

The Pedagogy of the Postcard: The invention and mass distribution of the picture postcard turned millions of everyday citizens into active participants in the dissemination of colonial imagery. Postcards featuring posed portraits of human exhibition captives were printed by the millions, mailed across continents, and collected in family albums, normalizing the objectification of non-Western peoples in private domestic spaces across the globe.

Chronological Milestones: The Turning Points That Shattered the Exhibition Era

The decline and ultimate collapse of the human exhibition industry did not happen overnight; it was punctuated by specific, high-profile historical events, controversies, and legal interventions that progressively stripped the practice of its cultural legitimacy:

The Ota Benga Controversy at the Bronx Zoo (September 1906): The display of Ota Benga, a young Mbuti (Congo) man, inside the Monkey House of the New York Zoological Park marked a critical moral flashpoint in the United States. Prompted by Black clergymen, led by James H. Gordon, public outrage erupted against zoo director William Hornaday. Though the exhibition lasted only days before Benga was removed to an asylum and later an orphanage, the national debate exposed the cruel intersection of scientific racism and public entertainment, forcing American institutions to tread more cautiously with live human displays.

The Communist Counter-Exhibition "The Truth on the Colonies" (Paris, 1931): Concurrently with the massive state-sponsored Paris Colonial Exposition of 1931—which drew tens of millions of visitors to view human village dioramas—the French Communist Party and anti-colonial intellectuals organized a sharp counter-exhibition titled La Vérité sur les Colonies. Though modest in attendance, this intellectual challenge utilized Marxist and early anti-imperialist frameworks to systematically dismantle the official rhetoric of the "civilizing mission," planting the seeds for postwar decolonization.

The Aftermath of World War II and the Universal Declaration of Human Rights (1948): The profound moral devastation of the Holocaust, combined with the active participation of colonial troops from Africa and Asia in defeating fascism, made the continued racial degradation of human exhibitions culturally untenable in Europe. The formal adoption of the United Nations Universal Declaration of Human Rights established an international legal standard that rendered the public caging and display of human beings an explicit violation of universal dignity.

The 1958 Brussels World's Fair (Expo 58) and the Final "Congolese Village": Widely recognized by historians as the last major international exposition to feature a human display, Expo 58 in Belgium included a reconstructed "Congolese village". However, unlike nineteenth-century exhibitions, the event faced intense scrutiny, organized protests from newly politicized Congolese students and visitors, and widespread embarrassment among Western organizers. The overwhelming cultural friction at Expo 58 signaled that the era of the human zoo was dead, closing the chapter on state-sanctioned human exhibitions.

The Closure of France's Last Reported Human Display (Port Saint-Père, September 1994): Proving that the ghost of the exhibition era lingered close to the modern threshold, a safari park in Port Saint-Père, France, recreated a "human village" featuring Ivorian musicians, dancers, and actors. Prompted by swift legal action from anti-racism coalitions such as No to the Human Zoo, the exhibit was forced to close. This milestone demonstrated that civil society remained permanently mobilized to extinguish any modern revival of colonial objectification.

The Aftershocks of 1958: The Institutional Awakening and Legal Bans

Following the intense cultural friction at the 1958 Brussels World's Fair, Western governments and international cultural organizations could no longer ignore the toxic incompatibility between modern human rights frameworks and live ethnographic displays. This realization triggered a wave of municipal ordinances, national legislation, and internal administrative directives that permanently outlawed the practice:

Municipal Code Revisions: Major European and American cities that had historically hosted world's fairs quietly updated their municipal event licensing codes, inserting explicit bans on the public exhibition of human beings within commercial, zoological, or fairground settings. Promoters who had previously relied on municipal cooperation found themselves facing immediate permit denials and severe penal sanctions.

The Shift in Anthropological Ethics: Professional anthropological associations worldwide—including the American Anthropological Association and the Société d'Anthropologie de Paris—issued formal condemnations of their own disciplinary histories. They instituted strict ethical charters prohibiting members from participating in, advising, or lending scientific credibility to any event that commodified cultural groups for public entertainment.

The Role of Decolonization Movements in Dismantling the Gaze

The rapid dismantling of human exhibitions was deeply accelerated by the global wave of decolonization that swept across Africa and Asia following the Second World War. As colonized nations fought for and won political independence, the geopolitical power imbalance that had permitted Western showmen to recruit or coerce performers evaporated:

Diplomatic Retaliation and Protests: Newly independent governments established immediate diplomatic oversight over foreign travel and cultural exchange. Embassies in London, Paris, Brussels, and Washington actively monitored and intervened against any commercial enterprise attempting to export citizens for exhibition abroad, treating such efforts as violations of national sovereignty and human dignity.

The Reversal of the Gaze: Decolonization fundamentally inverted the psychological power dynamic of the exhibition era. Instead of Western spectators gazing down upon colonized subjects within a European park, newly liberated nations hosted international conferences, cultural festivals, and sports events—such as the 1955 Bandung Conference—where non-Western peoples defined their own modernities, artistic achievements, and political futures on their own terms.

The Archival Silences and the Politics of Historical Redaction

As modern scholars attempt to reconstruct the full scope of the human exhibition era, they frequently encounter deliberate gaps, redactions, and destructions within municipal and corporate archives. The architecture of forgetting was not merely passive; it was often an active, administrative effort to sanitize the historical record:

Shredding the Ledger: Historical investigations into nineteenth- and twentieth-century exhibition companies reveal that many commercial promoters systematically destroyed their own employment contracts, medical logs, and correspondence records as public pressure mounted. Fearing legal liability, public censure, and criminal prosecution, these entities wiped clean the paper trails documenting the true conditions of captivity.

The Bureaucracy of Neutrality: Official government documents from the height of the colonial exhibition era frequently sanitized human suffering through clinical, bureaucratic euphemisms. Performers who died of exhaustion, malnutrition, or introduced European diseases were logged simply as "repatriated due to medical necessity" or "deceased of natural causes," obscuring the lethal reality of the fairground enclosures behind official administrative jargon.

The Intergenerational Trauma and Descendant Healing Rituals

The legacy of human zoos did not end with the physical demolition of the pavilions or the signing of municipal bans; it echoed deeply within the families and communities from which captives were taken. The psychological wounds of objectification, displacement, and unburied ancestors created generational ripples that required deliberate, community-led mechanisms of healing:

Reclaiming Ancestral Memory: Descendants of exhibition survivors have undertaken extensive grassroots genealogical projects to track down family members who vanished into the European and American fairground circuits. By piecing together fragments of letters, overseas shipping manifests, and archival photographs, families are successfully reclaiming the individual identities of those whom the exhibition industry tried to reduce to anonymous types.

Ceremonial Closure and Reburial: In recent years, indigenous and African communities have organized formal, spiritual ceremonies of return for ancestors whose remains were kept in university anatomy departments and museum vaults after dying in human zoos. These sacred rituals of reburial serve as a powerful counter-narrative to the public exhibition of the past, returning dignity, peace, and sacred rest to those who were denied it in life.

The Final Reckoning: Living in a Post-Exhibition World

The historical trajectory of the human exhibition era stands fully exposed: from its origins in imperial hubris and commercial greed to its painful unravelling under the weight of moral awakening, whistleblowing, and global decolonization. The world did not simply stop looking away by accident; it was forced to do so through the tireless labor of activists, the courage of surviving descendants, and an irreversible shift in international human rights consciousness.

The Permanent Sentinel of Memory: The closure of the final human displays and the ongoing repatriation of stolen remains and artifacts mark not an end to our responsibility, but a permanent baseline for modern ethics. The legacy of the human zoo serves as an enduring historical sentinel, warning modern society against the quiet return of objectification in media, tourism, and digital representation.

The Triumph of Inherent Dignity: Ultimately, history honors the resilience of the human spirit over the machinery of exploitation. By looking away from the false spectacles of the past and turning instead toward truth, accountability, and the restoration of voice, humanity took an essential step forward. The final verdict of history is clear: no culture, community, or individual can ever be reduced to a commodity for public consumption without violating the absolute, sacred dignity of the human soul.

Chapter 10

From Human Zoos to Human Rights

The Shadow of the Fairground on Modern Bioethics

The systemic exploitation, involuntary display, and unconsented medical measurement of human zoo captives did not vanish without a trace; rather, they are left deep, structural scars that fundamentally shaped the architecture of modern bioethics. During the nineteenth and early twentieth centuries, anthropologists, physicians, and exposition promoters routinely treated non-Western individuals as biological specimens rather than human subjects.

The Violation of Bodily Autonomy: Performers were frequently subjected to physical measurements, psychological testing, and post-mortem examinations without their knowledge or meaningful consent. The moral outrage generated by these medical and scientific abuses later served as a direct historical warning, informing the strict parameters of bodily autonomy that underpin contemporary medical ethics.

Rejecting the "Scientific" Justification: The legacy of human zoos dismantled the Victorian pretense that scientific inquiry could justify the suspension of basic human rights. Modern bioethical frameworks explicitly reject the utilitarian or pseudoscientific rationalizations that once permitted researchers to use marginalized populations as instruments for public spectacle or academic curiosity.

The Evolution of Informed Consent and Research Oversight

The transformation from institutional exploitation to rigorous research governance is directly linked to the historical reckoning over human exhibitions and colonial experimentation:

Codifying Consent: The principle of informed consent—mandating that human participants must fully understand, evaluate, and voluntarily agree to any study, display, or intervention—was forged in opposition to the deceptive recruitment tactics utilized by showmen and imperial researchers.

Institutional Review Boards (IRBs): Modern research ethics committees and institutional review boards trace their intellectual lineage to the collective realization that researchers and corporations cannot police their own ethical standards. The unchecked authority once granted fairground promoters and exposition directors demonstrated the vital necessity of independent, external oversight to protect vulnerable populations from coercion.

Museum Ethics and the Restorative Turn

The evolution of museum ethics in the late twentieth and twenty-first centuries represents a direct institutional response to the collecting practices of the human exhibition era:

Redefining the Institution's Purpose: Traditional ethnographic museums, once structured around the collection and display of exoticized "types," have undergone a profound philosophical revolution. Curatorial practices now prioritize collaboration with descendant communities, transparency of provenance, and the ethical stewardship of cultural heritage.

De-colonizing the Gallery Space: Modern Museum standards enforce strict protocols regarding human remains, sacred objects, and culturally sensitive artifacts. The institutional memory of human zoos acts as a permanent check against the temptation to sensationalize foreign cultures for attendance numbers, ensuring that education never crosses the line into objectification.

International Human Rights Principles and Non-Repetition

The transition from the era of human exhibitions to the codification of universal human rights represents one of the most significant shifts in global jurisprudence:

Establishing Universal Protections: International frameworks, such as the Universal Declaration of Human Rights and subsequent treaties protecting indigenous and minority populations, were drafted with a acute awareness of the systemic abuses of the colonial and exhibition eras. These legal instruments explicitly prohibit degrading treatment, forced displacement, and the commercial exploitation of human dignity.

The Legal Guarantee of Non-Repetition: By formally classifying historical human exhibitions as violations of fundamental human rights, international courts and tribunals ensure that states and private entities remain legally bound to the principle of non-repetition, anchoring the absolute prohibition of human display into global law.

The Legal Codification of Human Dignity: From Moral Outrage to Binding Law

The transition from nineteenth-century fairground exploitation to twentieth- and twenty-first-century international law required a profound philosophical shift—one that translated abstract moral revulsion into enforceable legal doctrines. As global institutions were rebuilt in the wake of world wars and decolonization movements, the architects of international law drew direct lessons from the structural abuses of the human exhibition era:

Enshrining Inherent Worth: Foundational human rights instruments were drafted to explicitly reject the racial hierarchies and utilitarian logic that had justified human zoos. By embedding the principle of inherent human dignity into international charters, global jurists ensured that no state, corporation, or scientific body could legally claim that a human being's status could be reduced to that of a specimen or a public spectacle.

The Criminalization of Degrading Treatment: International humanitarian law and human rights conventions evolved to categorize public humiliation, forced servitude, and unauthorized physical exhibitions not merely as civil infractions, but as severe violations of international law. This legal firewall dismantled the commercial incentives that had once fueled the global exhibition circuit.

The Transformation of Anthropological and Scientific Governance

The fields of anthropology, ethnography, and human biology underwent radical internal reformation in response to the ethical failures of their intellectual predecessors. The academic establishment was forced to confront how nineteenth-century science had provided the intellectual scaffolding for human zoos:

Internal Ethics Charters: Professional organizations, including the International Union of Anthropological and Ethnological Sciences, established binding ethical codes that explicitly forbid researchers from participating in, endorsing, or profiting from any form of cultural exoticization or non-consensual human display.

Community-Led Research Methodologies: Modern scientific inquiry mandates participatory action research, wherein source communities act as equal partners, co-designing studies, retaining veto power over data publication, and ensuring that research directly benefits the population being studied. This structural shift effectively locked the door against the extractive, voyeuristic methodologies of the past.

The Reform of Cultural Heritage Law and International Treaties

The legal protections that prevent any modern recurrence of the human exhibition era extend deep into the realm of international cultural heritage law. Recognizing that the commodification of human beings often began with the unauthorized seizure and trafficking of cultural artifacts and ancestral remains, global legislative bodies instituted strict international frameworks:

The UNESCO Conventions: International treaties, such as the 1970 UNESCO Convention on the Means of Prohibiting and Preventing the Illicit Import, Export and Transfer of Ownership of Cultural Property, established robust mechanisms to halt the transnational trafficking of stolen heritage. These legal instruments ensure that source nations and indigenous communities retain sovereign authority over their cultural patrimony, blocking the commercial networks that once fed museum and fairground collections alike.

Protection of Intangible Cultural Heritage: Beyond physical objects, modern international law protects living cultural expressions, oral traditions, and customary practices from commercial exploitation. UNESCO's Convention for the Safeguarding of the Intangible Cultural Heritage ensures that indigenous music, dance, ritual, and knowledge systems cannot be appropriated, distorted, or turned into unauthorized public spectacles without the explicit, free, and informed consent of the practitioners.

Institutional Accountability and the Rise of Ethical Curatorship

The historical reckoning of human zoos permanently transformed how public institutions curate, display, and interpret history for the modern citizen:

Transparent Provenance and Restitution: Museums and academic repositories worldwide have implemented rigorous provenance research programs to uncover the dark histories behind their holdings. When collections are found to have been acquired through colonial coercion, scientific theft, or fairground exploitation, institutions are increasingly expected to initiate proactive dialogue for repatriation and restitution.

Decentering the Colonial Voice: Modern curatorial ethics mandate collaborative curation, wherein descendant communities and historically marginalized groups write their own labels, design their own gallery spaces, and control their own narratives. This structural democratization of the museum space ensures that the voyeuristic gaze of the nineteenth-century exhibition is permanently replaced by self-representation, historical truth, and mutual respect.

The Intersection of Global Health Standards and Human Subject Protection

The legacy of human zoos and colonial medicine forged an indelible link between the exploitation of fairground captives and the evolution of international clinical research ethics. During the nineteenth and early twentieth centuries, physicians and biological researchers frequently utilized human exhibition venues and colonial outposts as testing grounds, operating entirely outside the boundaries of accountability:

The Nuremberg Code and Postwar Clinical Governance: The revelations of World War II atrocities forced the global medical community to codify strict protection for human subjects, culminating in the Nuremberg Code of 1947. This foundational text directly drew upon the historical trajectory of non-consensual human experimentation—roots that trace straight back to the medical examinations performed on human zoo captives without their understanding or agreement.

The Declaration of Helsinki: Developed by the World Medical Association, the Declaration of Helsinki further refined these principles, establishing that the well-being of the human subject must always take precedence over the interests of science and society. This ethical mandate permanently closed the door to utilitarian justifications that once allowed researchers to treat marginalized individuals as biological commodities for public or academic consumption.

The Rise of Corporate Accountability and Global Human Rights Compliance

As multinational corporations, entertainment conglomerates, and tourism giants operate on a truly global scale, the historical lessons of the human exhibition era continue to inform modern regulatory frameworks regarding corporate social responsibility:

Human Rights Due Diligence: Contemporary international standards, including the United Nations Guiding Principles on Business and Human Rights, require corporations to conduct rigorous due diligence to ensure their operations do not violate fundamental human dignity, exploit indigenous populations, or engage in cultural commodification.

Preventing Modern Spectacle Exploitation: Civil society organizations and international labor watchdogs apply the historical framework of human zoos to scrutinize modern forms of entertainment, reality television casting, and indigenous tourism. This constant vigilance ensures that the structural power imbalances of the past are actively identified, challenged, and prevented from re-emerging in the modern media and leisure economy.

The Architecture of Accountability: Legal Redress and Transitional Justice

As the global community confronts the multi-generational legacies of human exhibitions, the mechanisms of international human rights law have increasingly expanded to address historical grievances that were once deemed beyond the reach of the courts:

Expanding Legal Standing for Descendant Groups: Modern jurisprudence has progressively explored legal avenues for descendant communities to seek formal apologies, institutional reparations, and cultural restitution. By recognizing that the harm inflicted during the human exhibition era caused enduring social, psychological, and economic damage, legal scholars have built frameworks that bridge the gap between historical injustice and contemporary civil rights law.

Truth and Reconciliation Models: Drawing inspiration from transitional justice movements worldwide, cultural institutions and municipal governments have begun utilizing truth-telling commissions to formally document the local participation in human zoos. These official inquiries bring to light the municipal budgets, university involvement, and corporate profiteering that sustained the exhibitions, transforming hidden historical complicity into transparent public record.

The Permanent Legacy of Human Rights Education

The ultimate safeguard against any future iteration of human exhibitionism lies in the systematic integration of human rights education into global academic curricula:

Teaching the Mechanics of Dehumanization: Educational frameworks now challenge students to analyze the precise propaganda techniques, pseudoscientific rationales, and media loops that made human zoos culturally acceptable to ordinary citizens in the past. Understanding how a society could normalize such cruelty serves as an essential inoculation against modern forms of xenophobia, cultural stereotyping, and the commodification of human lives.

The Global Ethic of Inviolable Dignity: The transition from human zoos to universal human rights represents one of humanity's most crucial moral evolutions. The hard-won lessons of the fairground era live on as an active legal, ethical, and philosophical commitment: that human beings are subjects of inherent worth and sovereign dignity, never objects to be displayed, measured, or consumed.

The Protection of Indigenous Self-Determination in the Digital Age

As the architecture of global communication shifts into virtual and digital realms, the lessons forged from the historical abuses of human exhibitions provide vital guardrails for the protection of indigenous and marginalized communities online:

Combating Digital Voyeurism: Modern human rights frameworks increasingly address the unauthorized digital capture, uploading, and algorithmic commodification of indigenous imagery, sacred rituals, and traditional lifestyles by tourists, vloggers, and media corporations. These digital practices are recognized as modern echoes of the fairground lens, reducing living cultures into passive online entertainment without consent or compensation.

Sovereignty Over Virtual Representation: Indigenous data sovereignty initiatives ensure that communities retain legal and ethical control over how their histories, images, and cultural expressions are stored, shared, and monetized across global digital platforms. This digital self-determination acts as a contemporary firewall, preventing the exploitation of the human exhibition era from finding new life in the metaverse, social media algorithms, and artificial intelligence training datasets.

The Intersection of Global Health Standards and Human Subject Protection

The historical trauma of non-consensual medical examinations conducted on human zoo captives laid bare the urgent need for international oversight in scientific research. As modern biomedical ethics matured, regulatory bodies codified ironclad protections to ensure that vulnerable populations could never again be exploited for institutional prestige or academic curiosity:

The Evolution of Ethical Review Boards: Modern clinical and social science research requires multi-layered approval from institutional review boards, ensuring that every study involving human participants undergoes rigorous scrutiny regarding risk assessment, voluntary participation, and equitable benefit distribution.

Global Monitoring of Exploitative Practices: International health organizations maintain active surveillance protocols to prevent clinical trials from bypassing ethical standards in developing nations or marginalized communities, directly countering the historical precedent set by colonial-era anthropologists and physicians who operated without legal or moral constraints.

The Role of Public Memory and Memorialization

Ensuring that the lessons of the human exhibition era remain visible to future generations require deliberate acts of public architecture, historic designation, and artistic memorialization:

Markers of Conscience at Historical Sites: Cities that hosted major world fairs and human exhibitions have begun installing official historical markers, plaques, and commemorative monuments at the exact sites of former enclosures. These installations reject the whitewashed narratives of past civic boosters, educating the public on the dark realities that took place on those grounds.

Public Art as Restorative Dialogue: Contemporary sculptors, muralists, and installation artists are commissioned to create works that honor the resilience of those who were displayed, transforming spaces of historical humiliation into sites of reflection, education, and collective healing.

The Codification of Cultural Rights in International Jurisprudence

The legal evolution from the era of human exhibitions to contemporary international human rights law found its most sophisticated expression in the explicit protection of cultural rights. Recognizing that the destruction of a people's dignity often begins with the distortion and commercialization of their heritage, international bodies have established binding legal safeguards:

Cultural Self-Identification as a Fundamental Right: Modern international instruments, including the United Nations Declaration on the Rights of Indigenous Peoples (UNDRIP), enshrinement of the right of communities to define their own identities, traditions, and futures without external interference. This legal principle directly invalidates the patronizing logic of the nineteenth-century showman who claimed the authority to categorize and display human beings.

Prohibiting Forced Assimilation and Public Degradation: Contemporary human rights law explicitly outlaws state-sponsored or commercially driven policies of forced assimilation and cultural degradation. Practices that expose marginalized groups to public ridicule, voyeurism, or humiliation are classified under international conventions as severe affronts to human security and dignity.

The Ongoing Vigilance of Civil Society and Grassroots Coalitions

While international treaties and institutional reforms provide essential structural defenses, the ultimate guarantor of a post-exhibition world remains active civil society mobilization:

Community-Led Watchdog Organizations: Across the globe, grassroots networks, anti-racism coalitions, and cultural preservation societies operate as permanent sentinels against modern attempts to revive exoticized human displays. Whether intervening against unauthorized commercial village setups in theme parks or challenging exploitative media tropes, these organizations ensure that the hard-learned lessons of history are actively defended in daily public life.

The Permanent Duty of Remembrance: The transition from human zoos to universal human rights is an ongoing, active commitment. By maintaining institutional transparency, honoring ancestral memories, and fiercely protecting human dignity from commodification, the global community ensures that the world will never again look away from injustice.

The Intersection of Global Environmental and Cultural Rights

As international human rights law continues to evolve, the framework established in the wake of the human exhibition era has expanded to encompass the protection of indigenous lands, ecologies, and traditional knowledge systems:

Recognizing Ecocultural Interdependence: Modern jurisprudence increasingly acknowledges that the forced displacement of indigenous communities for colonial exhibitions was deeply intertwined with the theft of their ancestral lands. International declarations now link cultural survival directly to territorial integrity, ensuring that communities cannot be separated from their native habitats for economic exploitation, tourism, or public spectacle.

Safeguarding Traditional Ecological Knowledge: Global scientific and environmental bodies have implemented strict legal protocols to protect indigenous ecological expertise from corporate biopiracy and unauthorized appropriation. This prevents researchers and commercial enterprises from extracting traditional medicines and environmental practices without explicit consent, mirroring the legal reforms that ended the non-consensual biological measurement of human zoo captives.

The Role of Transnational Transitional Justice and Diplomatic Apologies

The modern reckoning with human exhibitions has entered the realm of official state diplomacy and transnational transitional justice, moving beyond domestic policy changes into formal international accountability:

State-Level Apologies and Historical Reckoning: Heads of state, municipal mayors, and parliamentary bodies in nations with histories of organizing human zoos have begun issuing formal, public apologies to descendant communities and source nations. These official acknowledgments validate decades of grassroots advocacy and establish an unalterable public record of historical state-sponsored abuse.

Bilateral Restitution Agreements: Beyond symbolic apologies, governments are increasingly establishing bilateral agreements to finance educational programs, support descendant genealogical research, and fund community-led memorial projects. These structured reparations transform abstract historical guilt into concrete acts of restorative justice, cementing the global standard that historical human rights violations demand tangible remediation.

The Reform of International Tourism Ethics and Fair Travel Standards

The legacy of human exhibitions profoundly shaped the modern critique of mass tourism, particularly the commodification of indigenous cultures through voyeuristic travel packages:

The Global Code of Ethics for Tourism: Adopted by the United Nations World Tourism Organization, international travel frameworks explicitly prohibit exploitative tourism models that treat living communities as tourist attractions or living museums. These standards mandate that cultural tourism must be based on mutual respect, sustainability, and the explicit consent of host populations.

Challenging "Human Safari" Enterprises: Civil society watchdogs and responsible travel coalitions actively monitor and shut down commercial operations that attempt to market indigenous villages as human dioramas. This ongoing oversight ensures that the travel industry adheres to the strict human rights boundaries established after the collapse of the fairground era.

The Codification of Rights in Post-Colonial Constitutions

The hard-won lessons of the human exhibition era left an indelible mark on the constitutional development of newly independent nations during the decolonization wave:

Constitutional Protections Against Degrading Treatment: Post-colonial states frequently embedded rigorous anti-discrimination and anti-degradation clauses into their foundational supreme laws, explicitly criminalizing any public act that violates human dignity or reduces citizens to objects of curiosity or racial ridicule.

Sovereign Control Over Cultural Export: These constitutional frameworks established absolute state and community sovereignty over the circulation of cultural heritage, performers, and artifacts abroad, ensuring that foreign governments and private enterprises could never again unilaterally export human beings for exhibition without strict legal authorization and oversight.

The Integration of Human Rights Standards into Corporate and Public Sector Procurement

As global institutions systematically align with post-colonial ethics, the strict principles forged in opposition to human exhibitions have penetrated modern procurement and operational guidelines:

Ethical Event and Exhibition Licensing: Municipalities and international organizations now enforce mandatory human rights compliance screenings for all contractors, festival organizers, and cultural event promoters. Any proposal that relies on exoticized human displays, ethnic stereotyping, or non-consensual cultural performance is instantly disqualified and barred from public funding or venue access.

Corporate Social Responsibility Audits: Major entertainment corporations, cruise lines, and media networks undergo mandatory third-party audits to ensure their cultural programming, shore excursions, and documentary practices strictly uphold indigenous self-determination and dignity, preventing any corporate regression toward fairground-era voyeurism.

The Role of International Human Rights Courts in Preventing Non-Repetition

The ultimate enforcement mechanism of modern human rights law lies within international judicial bodies, which treat any attempt to revive human exhibitionism as a direct violation of international jus cogens norms:

Precedents on Human Dignity and Autonomy: International courts and human rights tribunals have solidified legal precedents establishing that the right to human dignity is non-derogatable, meaning it can never be suspended for reasons of scientific curiosity, commercial entertainment, or state interest. This legal bedrock stands as a permanent barrier against the ideologies that enabled human zoos.

The Enforcement of Global Restitution Orders: Regional human rights courts increasingly possess the mandate to issue binding judgments requiring governments and public institutions to return stolen cultural heritage, fund commemorative sites, and enact legislative safeguards, ensuring that historical injustices are met with enforceable legal remediation.

The Evolution of Global Media Ethics and Self-Regulation

The transformation of media and broadcasting standards represents a critical frontier in preventing any modern recurrence of the human exhibition era. As mass media expanded through television, documentary film, and digital streaming, international regulatory bodies and journalistic organizations were forced to confront the persistent temptation to exoticize non-Western or marginalized communities:

Strict Broadcasting Codes and Consent Protocols: Modern public service and commercial broadcasting authorities enforce rigorous ethical guidelines that prohibit the exploitation, misrepresentation, or voyeuristic framing of vulnerable populations. Documentarians and reality television producers are legally and professionally mandated to secure informed consent, ensure fair compensation, and grant subjects review over their narrative portrayal.

Challenging Exoticizing Tropes: Media watchdog organizations continuously audit global entertainment output to dismantle persistent colonial tropes—such as portraying indigenous groups as "primitive" or "unchanged by time" for Western audience consumption. This active cultural critique ensures that modern media channels do not inadvertently replicate the psychological distancing and spectacle-driven logic of the nineteenth-century fairground.

The Intersection of Global Archives and Restorative Digital Repositories

As modern technology redefines how historical data is preserved and shared, the fight against the archival erasure of human zoo victims has entered the digital sphere:

Decentralized Digital Archives: International coalitions of historians, universities, and descendant communities are building secure, open-access digital repositories that aggregate fragmented records, photographs, and contracts from nineteenth-century exhibition companies. These platforms ensure that the identities, origins, and personal histories of captives cannot be hidden or destroyed by institutional gatekeepers.

Open-Source Provenance Tracking: Advanced digital tools allow researchers to trace the illicit movement of human remains and cultural artifacts across global museum networks in real time, streamlining the legal and administrative processes required for rightful repatriation and closure.

The Permanent Guardian of Global Ethics

The Living Blueprint of Human Rights: The transformation from the dark spectacles of human zoos to the universal protection of human rights stands as one of history's most critical civilizational shifts. The enduring legacy of this era serves as a permanent, active guardian—reminding global institutions, legal systems, and societies that human dignity is absolute, non-negotiable, and inviolable under any circumstances.

The Evolution of Human Rights Jurisprudence on Bodily Integrity

The legal legacy of human zoos extends deeply into the modern interpretation of bodily integrity as an absolute legal right. In the nineteenth and early twentieth centuries, fairgrounds and scientific expositions operated on the premise that marginalized bodies were public property, subject to inspection, measurement, and exhibition without permission:

The Prohibition of Biological Commodification: Modern international human rights law explicitly outlaws the commodification of the human body, drawing a direct legal line from the forced physical measurements of human zoo captives to contemporary prohibitions on human trafficking, forced organ harvesting, and unauthorized biological sampling.

Autonomy as a Universal Standard: Contemporary constitutional and international frameworks enshrine bodily autonomy as an unalienable right, guaranteeing that no individual can be compelled to submit to physical exhibition, medical intervention, or public display against their will, regardless of state mandate or commercial contract.

The Role of Public Historians and Memorialization Coalitions

The transition from hidden historical complicity to active public remembrance relies heavily on the work of contemporary public historians, educators, and memorial coalitions:

Rewriting Civic Narratives: Municipalities that once hosted colonial expositions are increasingly partnering with public historians to rewrite official guidebooks, exhibition catalogs, and museum plaques. This active correction ensures that the historical record reflects the exploitation, coercion, and resistance of those who were exhibited, rather than the self-congratulatory myths of nineteenth-century civic boosters.

Global Networks of Conscience: International coalitions of museums, human rights organizations, and descendant groups now collaborate to share best practices in historical reckoning, ensuring that the dark chapters of human display are taught transparently across educational systems worldwide.

The Reform of International Intellectual Property and Folklore Protections

The historical exploitation of human zoos frequently relied on the unauthorized theft, parody, and commercialization of indigenous songs, dances, clothing, and spiritual rituals. This extraction laid the groundwork for modern debates over cultural property:

Securing Intellectual Property for Traditional Arts: Modern legal frameworks, spearheaded by the World Intellectual Property Organization (WIPO), have developed specialized instruments to protect traditional cultural expressions (TCEs) from commercial misappropriation. These mechanisms prevent outside corporations and entertainers from patenting or profiting from indigenous designs, music, and folklore without the consent of the culture bearers.

Ending Cultural Misappropriation in Commercial Media: International standards hold media companies and entertainment producers legally accountable for the unauthorized replication of sacred or culturally specific practices. This creates a powerful deterrent against the modern revival of exoticized, fairground-style tropes in global cinema, fashion, and advertising.

The Role of Youth Education and Global Civic Curricula

To ensure that the hard-won lessons of the human exhibition era endure across generations, educational reformers have integrated the history of human zoos into civic and human rights curricula worldwide:

Critical Media Literacy as a Defense: Modern educational standards teach students how to identify exoticization, dehumanization, and orientalist tropes in historical and contemporary media. By analyzing the propaganda techniques used by nineteenth-century exhibition promoters, students develop a critical lens against modern forms of xenophobia and cultural voyeurism.

Empathy and Global Citizenship: Curricula that address the human zoo era emphasize empathy, mutual respect, and the absolute equality of all human cultures. This pedagogical shift replaces outdated colonial narratives with a global ethic of universal human dignity, ensuring that the historical memory of these abuses actively safeguards future human rights.

The Intersection of Artificial Intelligence and Ethical Representation

As advanced machine learning and generative artificial intelligence reshape global media and cultural production, the historical lessons of human exhibitions provide vital ethical guardrails against digital exploitation:

Preventing Algorithmic Exoticization: Modern artificial intelligence governance frameworks explicitly target the generation of biased, stereotypical, or exoticized digital avatars and synthetic media. International regulatory bodies apply the anti-exploitation principles born from the human zoo era to ensure that AI models do not autonomously reproduce colonial tropes, cultural caricatures, or non-consensual digital reconstructions of marginalized groups.

Consent in Synthetic Media and Digital Cloning: Contemporary digital rights legislation mandates strict consent protocols regarding the scanning, replication, and virtual performance of human likenesses. This legal standard prevents media corporations and technology platforms from turning digital representations of living or historical individuals into passive spectacles for commercial consumption, effectively modernizing the fight against unauthorized human display.

The Transnational Solidarity of Descendant Communities

The modern global movement against the legacy of human exhibitions is anchored by the powerful cross-border solidarity of descendant networks:

Cross-Border Activism and Resource Sharing: Descendant communities from Africa, Asia, the Americas, and the Pacific have established robust international coalitions to support one another in archival research, legal restitution claims, and the public reframing of history. This transnational unity amplifies local advocacy into a global force for restorative justice.

The Permanent Global Standard of Inviolable Worth: The long journey from the dark exhibition tents of the nineteenth century to the sophisticated human rights architectures of the modern era stands as proof that collective memory, legal vigilance, and moral clarity can permanently reshape civilization. The foundational principle remains clear: human beings are subjects of absolute dignity, never objects to be displayed.

The Legal Evolution of Consent in Global Entertainment and Performance Law

The legacy of human zoos fundamentally reshaped modern entertainment law, transforming the legal baseline for consent, labor rights, and performance contracts involving human subjects:

The Abolition of Indentured Performance Contracts: Nineteenth-century exhibition companies frequently relied on deceptive, coercive, or unreadable contracts to bind foreign performers on long-term tours under abusive conditions. Modern labor laws and international entertainment standards strictly invalidate any contract that lacks informed consent, fair compensation, or guarantees of safe, voluntary repatriation.

Special Protections for Traveling Performers and Troupes: Contemporary labor jurisdictions enforce rigorous oversight on international cultural troupes, circuses, and performance collectives, ensuring that foreign artists are treated as autonomous professionals rather than exoticized commodities. This legal shield directly dismantles the structural power imbalances that once allowed showmen to exploit human beings as fairground attractions.

The Role of Museum Ethics Codes in Global Curatorial Practice

As the institutional legacy of human exhibitions continues to face rigorous public scrutiny, professional museum associations worldwide have codified binding ethical standards to prevent any repetition of past abuses:

International Council of Museums (ICOM) Guidelines: Modern ethical codes explicitly prohibit museums from acquiring, displaying, or retaining human remains or cultural objects acquired through colonial coercion, scientific theft, or exhibition exploitation. These guidelines mandate proactive transparency, strict provenance verification, and open communication with descendant communities.

Deaccessioning and Ethical Governance: Museums are increasingly utilizing ethical deaccessioning frameworks to return contested holdings to their rightful owners or source nations. This institutional shift ensures that public repositories function as spaces of education, truth, and mutual respect rather than storehouses for the spoils of nineteenth-century imperialism.

The Intersection of Global Trade Policy and Cultural Artifact Protection

The movement to dismantle the lingering infrastructure of human exhibitions has increasingly intersected with international trade policy and intellectual property treaties, creating robust economic defenses against cultural exploitation:

Trade Sanctions on Illicit Cultural Trafficking: International trade agreements now incorporate strict enforcement mechanisms penalizing the commercial smuggling of human remains, sacred relics, and historical documents associated with colonial exploitation and human zoos. Customs agencies worldwide are empowered to seize and repatriate contested objects before they reach private auction houses or commercial markets.

Binding Cultural Protections in Free Trade Agreements: Modern bilateral and multilateral trade pacts frequently include explicit exemptions for indigenous cultural heritage. These clauses ensure that international commerce cannot override local sovereignty laws or force nations to open their cultural expressions to unregulated commercialization and foreign exploitation.

The Role of Municipal Public History and Urban Planning in Reparations

As cities across Europe, the Americas, and beyond confront their direct municipal involvement in organizing nineteenth-century world fairs and colonial expositions, urban planning has become an active medium for restorative justice:

De-Colonizing Public Space and Infrastructure: Municipal governments are systematically renaming streets, parks, and public squares that historically honored the promoters, showmen, and politicians behind human zoos, replacing them with designations honoring resistance leaders and victims of colonial abuse.

Civic Investment in Descendant Communities: Forward-thinking urban planning now pairs historical markers with targeted civic investments, directing public funds toward educational infrastructure, cultural centers, and economic development programs in marginalized communities disproportionately impacted by historical human exhibitionism.

The Reform of International Documentary and Media Ethics

The voyeuristic techniques perfected during the human exhibition era left a profound legacy on early cinema, photography, and documentary filmmaking, where marginalized populations were routinely framed as exotic spectacles for Western audiences. In response, modern media ethics has undergone a sweeping transformation to eliminate these exploitative practices:

Informed Consent and Collaborative Storytelling: Modern documentary standards mandate that filmmakers secure explicit, informed consent from all participants, shifting the paradigm from observational voyeurism to collaborative storytelling. Subjects are no longer treated as passive objects of study or entertainment, but as active co-creators who retain editorial agencies over how their lives and cultures are depicted.

Prohibiting Poverty Pornography and Exoticized Framing: International journalistic and broadcasting bodies have established strict ethical guidelines against poverty porn and the deliberate distortion of foreign cultures for dramatic effect. These regulations directly dismantle the visual vocabulary of the nineteenth-century fairground, ensuring that modern media respects the comprehensive human dignity of every community it portrays.

The Codification of Universal Human Rights in Regional Legal Frameworks

The foundational principle that human beings can never be reduced to objects of exhibition or commercial display has been formally integrated into the statutory frameworks of regional human rights systems across the globe:

The Inter-American and European Human Rights Systems: Landmark rulings by regional courts have established strict judicial doctrines affirming that public degradation, racial stereotyping, and violations of cultural autonomy constitute severe breaches of fundamental human rights. These rulings provide binding legal precedents that protect vulnerable populations from state or commercial exploitation.

Transnational Enforcement of Dignity Protections: Regional human rights commissions maintain active monitoring mechanisms to investigate complaints regarding the commercial misappropriation of indigenous identity, unauthorized public displays, and cultural degradation, ensuring that the hard-won legal protections against human zoos are rigorously upheld across international borders.

The Intersection of Global Migration and Refugee Protection

The dismantling of nineteenth-century human exhibition structures fundamentally reconfigured modern international law regarding human displacement, asylum, and cross-border mobility. Early human zoos routinely relied on the imperial seizure, trafficking, and forced detention of displaced populations, treating refugees and colonized subjects as legally unprotected commodities available for public amusement. In direct opposition to this legacy, contemporary refugee law and international humanitarian conventions establish that displaced persons retain full legal personhood, bodily autonomy, and freedom from arbitrary detention. Modern asylum frameworks explicitly recognize that fleeing war, famine, or persecution does not strip individuals of their fundamental dignity or reduce them to spectacles of state charity. By binding nations to strict non-refoulement principles and mandating humane reception standards, international jurisprudence ensures that the vulnerable migrant is treated as a bearer of inviolable human rights rather than an object of curiosity or administrative voyeurism.

The Reform of Public Museum Anthropology and Display Ethics

Beyond the restitution of human remains and cultural artifacts, the contemporary museum landscape has undergone a profound structural revolution in how anthropology and human diversity are communicated to the public. Historically, anthropological museums functioned as permanent academic extensions of human zoos, utilizing pseudoscientific typologies, racial hierarchies, and static dioramas to freeze living cultures into primitive, archaic pasts. Today, modern curatorial ethics replace these colonial frameworks with participatory museology, wherein source communities actively co-author exhibition narratives, control the interpretation of their own histories, and dictate the terms on which their heritage is shared. This paradigm shift eradicates the vestige of the exhibitionary gaze, transforming public institutions from colonial cabinets of curiosities into dynamic spaces of cross-cultural dialogue, historical accountability, and mutual respect.

The Architecture of Global Architectural Memorialization and Healing Spaces

The physical reconstruction of historical memory has increasingly materialized through intentional architecture and landscape design, transforming the urban topology of former colonial capitals into sites of profound moral reflection. Architects and urban planners collaborating with descendant communities now conceptualize memorial spaces not merely as passive markers of past atrocities, but as active centers for civic education and restorative justice. These environments intentionally reject the monumentalism of nineteenth-century imperial architecture—which glorified state expansion and human subjugation—in favor of subterranean galleries, reflective reflection pools, and open-air forums designed to center the voices, names, and agency of those who suffered inside exhibition enclosures. By embedding these sites of conscience into the urban fabric, cities foster an ongoing public dialogue that counters historical amnesia and reinforces the spatial permanence of human dignity.

The Codification of Corporate Accountability in Transnational Supply Chains

The ideological shift away from human exhibitionism has fundamentally transformed contemporary corporate governance, particularly regarding multinational enterprises operating within regions historically impacted by imperial exploitation. Modern international business guidelines, such as the United Nations Guiding Principles on Business and Human Rights, mandate that corporations conduct rigorous human rights due diligence to ensure their operations do not replicate the coercive labor practices, cultural appropriations, or dignity violations characteristic of colonial enterprise. Companies are legally and ethically obligated to identify, prevent, and mitigate any adverse impacts on local populations, ensuring that global commerce respects indigenous self-determination and labor autonomy. This corporate accountability framework establishes that economic globalization must operate under the strict rule of universal human rights, permanently barring any commercial enterprise from treating human communities as disposable labor or passive spectacles.

The Intersection of Global Sports Diplomacy and Ethical Event Governance

The modern regulation of international athletic competitions and global sporting mega-events bears a direct lineage to the reform movements that dismantled nineteenth-century human exhibitions. Historically, colonial expositions frequently integrated athletic contests, native games, and physical demonstrations into human zoos, forcing indigenous athletes to perform as exoticized spectacles rather than recognized professional competitors. In response, modern sports governance bodies—such as the International Olympic Committee and global athletic federations—have established rigorous human rights requirements for host nation selection and event management. These protocols mandate strict anti-discrimination policies, fair labor standards for stadium construction, and the absolute protection of cultural autonomy for participating delegations. By enforcing these standards, international sport has transitioned from a historical extension of colonial fairground display into a platform for national sovereignty, mutual respect, and universal athletic equality.

The Role of Transnational Truth Commissions in Historic Injustice

As global mechanisms for transitional justice have matured, truth and reconciliation commissions have increasingly expanded their remits to investigate state-sponsored human exhibitions, colonial scientific experimentation, and the forced transnational trafficking of human subjects. Unlike conventional criminal tribunals, these commissions provide a specialized platform for descendant communities to testify regarding the generational trauma, archival erasure, and dignity violations inflicted by historical human zoos. The public testimony gathered by these bodies results in comprehensive state archives, official historical findings, and policy recommendations that guide legislative reparations, educational reforms, and institutional decolonization. This formal investigative process ensures that the atrocities of the human exhibition era are fully documented, legally recognized, and integrated into the permanent historical consciousness of modern nation-states.

The Reform of International Public Health Ethics and Pandemic Governance

The historical intersection of public health policy and human exhibitions revealed some of the most severe abuses of the colonial era, during which physicians and anthropologists frequently utilized fairground captives for non-consensual medical experiments, biometric cataloging, and quarantine justification under the guise of epidemiological study. In response to this dark precedent, contemporary international health law and global pandemic governance frameworks have established uncompromising ethical boundaries. The World Health Organization and international bioethics treaties mandate that all public health interventions, clinical research programs, and cross-border medical responses must strictly prioritize individual consent, bodily autonomy, and equity. This modern architecture ensures that health emergencies can never be weaponized by states or institutions to justify the forced isolation, biomedical tracking, or public exposure of marginalized populations, anchoring global health policy in the absolute protection of human dignity.

The Role of Transnational Indigenous Diplomacy in Global Policymaking

The modern global consensus against human exhibitionism has been heavily propelled by the rise of organized transnational indigenous diplomacy, transforming those once targeted by colonial showmen into influential architects of international law. Through permanent forums at the United Nations and global human rights coalitions, indigenous leaders and descendant networks actively shape treaties concerning cultural heritage, traditional knowledge, and self-determination. This diplomatic empowerment ensures that international standards regarding human dignity and cultural preservation are continually updated to address emerging global challenges. By shifting from passive subjects of historical display to active authors of international jurisprudence, descendant communities have cemented a permanent global standard that guarantees human diversity is protected, respected, and self-defined across every tier of civil society.

The Intersection of Global Climate Justice and Indigenous Territorial Rights

The modern expansion of international human rights law has forged an undeniable link between the legacy of colonial human exhibitions and contemporary climate justice. Nineteenth-century human zoos operated alongside the forced territorial displacement of indigenous populations to clear land for imperial resource extraction and agricultural plantations. Today, international environmental frameworks increasingly recognize that the physical survival and cultural autonomy of descendant communities are entirely inseparable from their ancestral lands. Modern climate policy frameworks mandate that environmental conservation, green energy transitions, and carbon offset projects cannot proceed without the free, prior, and informed consent (FPIC) of indigenous populations. This legal standard prevents governments and corporations from repeating historical displacement patterns under the guise of ecological necessity, ensuring that land stewardship remains firmly in the hands of the communities who have protected those ecosystems for generations.

The Codification of Dignity in Post-Conflict Reconstruction and Peacebuilding

The institutional lessons derived from the dismantling of human exhibitionism have profoundly influenced modern post-conflict reconstruction and international peacebuilding mandates.

When nations rebuild following civil wars or authoritarian regimes, international peacebuilding frameworks now prioritize the restoration of cultural dignity, public truth-telling, and the dismantling of structural discrimination as core components of sustainable peace. Drawing directly from the anti-degradation principles established in human rights jurisprudence, contemporary peace accords explicitly prohibit state-sanctioned propaganda that relies on ethnic stereotyping, public humiliation, or the dehumanization of minority groups. By embedding these safeguards into transitional governance, the international community ensures that post-conflict societies build institutional cultures rooted in absolute equality, preventing the ideological resurgence of the exclusionary, exhibitionary mindset that once justified human zoos.

The Worldwide Harmonization of Global Bioethics and Transnational Research Governance

The international Health Architecture has achieved a profound global consensus regarding human subject protection, drawing direct lessons from the non-consensual physiological measurements and biomedical exploitation that characterized nineteenth-century human zoos. Multilateral institutions, including the World Health Organization (WHO) and the United Nations Educational, Scientific and Cultural Organization (UNESCO), have established universal bioethical standards that apply across all sovereign borders. These frameworks mandate that any cross-border medical research or anthropological study conducted in developing nations or among marginalized indigenous populations must secure transparent, community-level consent and undergo rigorous independent ethical review. By creating a unified global jurisdiction against biomedical commodification, these regulatory instruments ensure that no nation or scientific institution can bypass basic human rights protections under the pretext of academic inquiry or medical progress.

The Transnational Coalition of Global South and Indigenous Peoples' Forums

The global movement to dismantle the lingering ideological structures of colonial human exhibitions has been powerfully institutionalized through multinational coalitions uniting the Global South and indigenous peoples' networks worldwide. Operating across international summits, the Permanent Forum on Indigenous Issues, and global human rights tribunals, these unified alliances challenge systemic cultural erasure and advocate for binding international conventions on heritage protection. This transnational solidarity effectively shifts global policy formulation away from Eurocentric historical interpretations, ensuring that the collective memory of human zoos and imperial exploitation informs contemporary geopolitical standards. Through this worldwide cooperative framework, nations across Africa, Asia, the Americas, and the Pacific actively collaborate to enforce absolute global accountability, cementing human dignity as an uncompromisable foundation of international law.

The Worldwide Protection of Intangible Cultural Heritage in International Law

The global campaign against the legacy of human exhibitions has catalyzed a worldwide legal transformation regarding the safeguarding of intangible cultural heritage. Historically, human zoos relied on the unauthorized public performance, decontextualization, and mockery of living cultural traditions, treating sacred rituals, oral histories, and traditional music as public entertainment. In response, the international community, UNESCO's Convention for the Safeguarding of the Intangible Cultural Heritage—has established a comprehensive global framework that grants communities absolute ownership over their living traditions. This worldwide standard legally empowers indigenous populations and minority groups across every continent to control, restrict, or license the public presentation of their cultural expressions, effectively criminalizing the commercial voyeurism and cultural extraction that defined the fairground era.

The Transnational Accountability of Global Digital Platforms and Information Ecosystems

As information and communication technologies span the globe, international human rights frameworks are increasingly brought to bear on digital corporations to prevent the online resurgence of exoticized human displays and colonial tropes. Global coalitions of civil society organizations and international regulatory bodies now pressure transnational tech platforms to adopt strict content moderation policies that penalize digital human safaris, exploitative vlogging, and the non-consensual algorithmic distribution of indigenous imagery. By treating digital platforms as accountable participants in the global information ecosystem, international law ensures that the anti-exploitation principles born from the dismantling of human zoos are actively enforced across virtual borders, safeguarding human dignity in the digital age worldwide.

The Worldwide Transformation of Global Humanitarian Law and Civilian Protection

The historical evolution from human exhibitions to universal human rights has profoundly reshaped global humanitarian law, particularly concerning the legal protections afforded to civilian populations during international and internal armed conflicts. During the nineteenth and early twentieth centuries, imperial military campaigns frequently captured foreign combatants and non-combatants alike, transporting them back to metropolitan capitals to be exhibited in colonial expositions as living trophies of military conquest. In stark contrast, modern international humanitarian law—anchored by the Geneva Conventions and additional protocols—strictly prohibits the public display, humiliation, degradation, and instrumentalization of prisoners of war or civilian detainees. Global monitoring bodies enforce these protections globally, ensuring that individuals caught in zones of conflict are treated with absolute humanitarian respect, shielding them from the voyeuristic spectacles and wartime exploitation that characterized the height of the imperial exhibition era.

The Transnational Harmonization of Global Intellectual Property and Traditional Knowledge Treaties

The global safeguarding of indigenous intellectual property has reached unprecedented levels of international harmonization, directly addressing the legacy of human zoos where traditional designs, clothing, and spiritual artifacts were systematically looted, copied, and commercialized without authorization. Multilateral bodies, including the World Intellectual Property Organization (WIPO), have advanced binding international instruments that protect traditional knowledge (TK) and traditional cultural expressions (TCEs) from unauthorized transnational appropriation.

These global legal frameworks empower source communities across every continent to legally challenge corporations, fashion houses, and entertainment entities that attempt to profit from sacred cultural symbols. By enforcing these rigorous worldwide standards, the international community ensures that global commerce respects indigenous ownership, permanently closing the commercial avenues that once allowed fairground promoters to exploit native culture with impunity.

The Worldwide Eradication of Colonial Education and Curricular Decolonization

The global movement to dismantle the legacy of human exhibitions has catalyzed a comprehensive, worldwide reform of educational curricula, replacing Eurocentric colonial narratives with universal human rights standards. Historically, imperial school systems utilized photographs, dioramas, and pseudo-anthropological texts derived from human zoos to indoctrinate students with racist ideologies of European supremacy and civilizational hierarchy. Today, international educational coalitions and post-colonial ministries of education across Africa, Asia, the Americas, and Europe have instituted rigorous curricular decolonization mandates. These educational frameworks require schools to critically examine the history of human display, institutional racism, and imperial exploitation, ensuring that generations worldwide are grounded in an ethic of global citizenship, cultural equity, and mutual respect.

The Transnational Harmonization of Global Labor Standards and Anti-Trafficking Conventions

The operational blueprint of nineteenth-century human zoos—which relied on the deception, coercion, and transnational trafficking of foreign performers under bonded labor conditions—has been systematically dismantled by modern international labor and anti-trafficking law. Multilateral institutions such as the

International Labour Organization (ILO) and global anti-trafficking conventions enforce strict extraterritorial oversight on international performance troupes, cultural exchange programs, and migrant labor markets. These global legal frameworks mandate absolute freedom of movement, fair wages, voluntary repatriation rights, and informed consent for all traveling artists and workers. By binding sovereign nations to these universal labor protections, the international community ensures that the structural vulnerabilities exploited by historical showmen can no longer be leveraged for commercial entertainment or forced exhibition anywhere in the world.

The Worldwide Accountability of Global Financial Institutions and Development Banks

The global reckoning with the legacy of human exhibitions has increasingly penetrated the operational policies of multilateral development banks and international financial institutions. Historically, colonial expansion and imperial exhibitions were financed by capital investments that ignored indigenous rights, displaced local communities, and commodified natural and human resources for metropolitan profit. In direct response to this history, major global financial bodies—including the World Bank and regional development banks—have instituted mandatory environmental and social safeguard policies. These binding frameworks require comprehensive free, prior, and informed consent (FPIC) from indigenous and marginalized populations before any international capital can fund infrastructure projects, agricultural expansions, or tourism developments in vulnerable regions. By conditioning global financial assistance on strict human rights compliance and community self-determination, the international monetary system actively prevents the economic replication of colonial exploitation.

The Transnational Harmonization of Global Urban Memorialization and Counter-Monumentalism

The global movement to repair the spatial legacy of human zoos has manifested through a worldwide wave of counter-monumentalism and urban restorative planning. Cities across Europe, the Americas, Africa, and the Pacific that once hosted massive colonial expositions and human exhibitions are systematically transform their urban landscapes through transnational collaboration among public historians, urban planners, and descendant networks. This global shift moves beyond the mere removal of statues honoring colonial showmen and fairground promoters; it establishes international networks of "Sites of Conscience" that share best practices in public truth-telling, commemorative architecture, and community-led restorative projects. By aligning urban planning with universal human rights standards, municipalities worldwide ensure that public spaces function as active environments for historical education, cross-cultural healing, and the permanent affirmation of human dignity.

The Worldwide Proliferation of Truth, Reconciliation, and Restorative Justice Commissions

The global transition from the historical era of human exhibitions to contemporary universal human rights has increasingly relied on transnational truth and reconciliation mechanisms to address lingering historical trauma. Governments across multiple continents that previously organized or sanctioned colonial expositions and human zoos have established formal national commissions to investigate the systemic extraction, confinement, and public degradation of human subjects. These bodies provide a vital global forum for descendant communities to document archival erasures, trace missing ancestral remains, and establish unalterable historical records of state-sponsored exploitation. By institutionalizing public testimony and historical accountability, these commissions transform abstract historical guilt into active restorative justice, ensuring that the foundational abuses of the exhibition era are formally recognized and legally addressed on a global scale.

The Transnational Enforcement of Universal Jurisdiction for Cultural and Human Dignity Violations

The ultimate legal fortification against any resurgence of human exhibitionism lies within the expanding doctrine of universal jurisdiction in international criminal and human rights law. Modern legal scholarship and international tribunals increasingly recognize that severe violations of human dignity—such as human trafficking for public exhibition, forced cultural degradation, and the unauthorized commercial commodification of vulnerable populations—constitute gross breaches of international jus cogens norms. This legal framework empowers international and domestic courts to prosecute perpetrators of modern trafficking, forced display, and cultural exploitation regardless of where the offenses occurred. By establishing that the core protections against human zoos are universally binding across all sovereign states, the international community ensures an unyielding legal defense of human autonomy and absolute dignity worldwide.

The Ultimate Legacy of Human Dignity and the Unfinished Global Imperative

The dark spectacles of the fairground era—which weaponized pseudo-scientific racism, imperial conquest, and state-sanctioned voyeurism for public entertainment—laid bare the catastrophic depths to which human societies can sink when the inherent dignity of vulnerable populations is stripped away for profit and prestige.

In response to these historical atrocities, the modern global community has constructed an interconnected web of international law, bioethical oversight, cultural preservation treaties, digital rights protections, and transitional justice mechanisms. From the decolonization of museum curation and urban architecture to the rigorous enforcement of informed consent in media, scientific research, and global commerce, these institutional safeguards serve as an unyielding firewall against any resurgence of human exploitation.

Ultimately, this chapter serves as both a historical accounting and a living blueprint for the future. It reminds global institutions, legal systems, and civil societies worldwide that human rights are not static privileges granted by states, but absolute, inviolable baselines of human worth. By maintaining institutional transparency, honoring ancestral memory, and fiercely defending cultural self-determination across every digital, physical, and geopolitical frontier, the global community ensures that humanity will never again look away from injustice, cementing the absolute truth that every human being is an autonomous subject of infinite dignity, never an object to be displayed.

Chapter 11

A Nurse's Reflection

The Historical Echoes in Modern Healthcare

As today's nurses and healthcare professionals navigate increasingly complex clinical environments, the dark legacy of human exhibitions and colonial medical exploitation offers profound, sobering lessons. The historical practices of nineteenth-century human zoos—where vulnerable human beings were subjected to non-consensual examinations, public humiliation, and physiological measurement for institutional prestige—were frequently facilitated by physicians and scientific institutions that abandoned their ethical boundaries.

Today's clinicians must recognize that the foundational roots of modern medical racism, institutional paternalism, and patient commodification are deeply entangled with this history. By confronting these past abuses, contemporary healthcare providers gain critical awareness of how historical trauma continues to impact marginalized communities, shaping modern disparities in health outcomes, systemic mistrust, and healthcare accessibility.

Clinical Advocacy as a Professional Imperative

Rooted in the lessons of an era where human subjects were stripped of their voice and agency, modern nursing advocacy demands active intervention against systemic inequities and institutional indifference. Nurses serve as the primary guardians of patient welfare at the bedside, positioning them to challenge implicit bias, address social determinants of health, and protect patients from institutional coercion or administrative overreach. Effective advocacy requires moving beyond passive empathy to actively dismantle clinical practices that marginalize vulnerable populations, ensuring that every patient receives equitable, high-quality care regardless of race, socioeconomic status, or cultural background. By championing patient rights and institutional transparency, nurses ensure that the historical power imbalances of the exhibition era are systematically replaced by an uncompromising commitment to patient-centered justice.

Cultivating Cultural Humility and Anti-Racist Practice

The transition from colonial anthropology to modern healthcare demands a shift from rigid cultural competence to lifelong cultural humility. While cultural competence often implies a static checklist of traits associated with specific groups, cultural humility requires nurses to engage in continuous self-reflection, acknowledge their own positional power, and recognize patients as the ultimate authorities on their own lived experiences. In clinical practice, this means actively listening to indigenous and minority patients, validating historical and generational trauma, and eliminating stereotypical assumptions that can compromise medical decision-making. By practicing cultural humility, nurses dismantle the remnants of the exoticizing gaze, fostering clinical environments where diversity is respected, cultural autonomy is preserved, and every patient is seen as a fully complex individual.

Trauma-Informed Care and the Restoration of Bodily Autonomy

The physical and psychological trauma inflicted upon captives in historical human exhibitions underscores the absolute necessity of trauma-informed care in contemporary clinical practice. Trauma-informed nursing recognizes the pervasive impact of historical, systemic, and individual trauma, reshaping clinical workflows to prioritize physical safety, emotional trust, and collaborative decision-making. Nurses operate this framework by practicing radical informed consent, ensuring patients fully understand and control every aspect of their physical examination, diagnostic testing, and treatment plan. By honoring bodily autonomy and treating the patient as an active co-creator in their healthcare journey, nurses actively counteract the history of bodily commodification, ensuring that the clinical space remains a sanctuary of healing, dignity, and absolute human respect.

Interprofessional Collaboration and Systemic Accountability

The prevention of medical exploitation and the safeguarding of patient dignity cannot rest solely on individual bedside nurses;

they require a coordinated, interprofessional commitment across the entire healthcare system. Historically, the unethical display and examination of human subjects succeeded because institutional hierarchies shielded physicians and administrators from ethical accountability. Today's healthcare professionals must actively dismantle rigid, top-down institutional cultures that discourage the reporting of safety violations, discrimination, or ethical breaches.

By fostering collaborative environments where nurses, physicians, pharmacists, and social workers operate as equal partners in patient advocacy, healthcare systems establish robust internal watchdogs. This collective accountability ensures that ethical standards are universally enforced, preventing any institutional drift toward patient commodification and reinforcing the principle that hospital environments must prioritize human healing over administrative or academic convenience.

The Role of Reflective Practice and Continuous Ethical Vigilance

True professional transformation requires nurses to engage in rigorous, ongoing self-assessment regarding their own unconscious biases, institutional privileges, and clinical habits. The historical legacy of colonial medicine demonstrates how easily well-intentioned professionals can become complicit in systemic harm when they fail to critically examine their worldview. Contemporary nursing education and clinical leadership must cultivate continuous ethical vigilance, encouraging nurses to question routine practices that may inadvertently alienate, marginalize, or disempower patients. By treating ethical reflection as a vital, daily clinical tool rather than a passive academic concept, nurses ensure that the hard-won lessons of historical human rights movements are actively translated into compassionate, equitable, and transformative bedside care.

Navigating Health Inequities and the Social Determinants of Health

The legacy of colonial exploitation extends directly into contemporary public health disparities, where marginalized populations experience disproportionate burdens of chronic illness, inadequate healthcare access, and environmental injustices. Modern nurses are uniquely positioned on the front lines of community and acute care to identify how structural racism and historical marginalization manifest as preventable health crises. Effective nursing practice requires looking beyond immediate clinical symptoms to assess and address the social determinants of health—such as housing stability, food security, economic opportunity, and environmental safety. By engaging in community-level health promotion and advocating for equitable resource distribution, nurses help dismantle the structural barriers that continue to leave vulnerable communities exposed to systemic health disparities.

The Ethical Imperative of Pain Management and Empathetic Validation

Historical human exhibitions and colonial medical practices frequently relied on the dehumanizing myth that marginalized populations possessed a higher pain tolerance or lacked the same emotional capacity for suffering as dominant groups. Shockingly, the remnants of these false racialized assumptions can still subtly infiltrate modern clinical settings, contributing to well-documented disparities in pain assessment and analgesic administration. Today's nurses must maintain rigorous self-awareness to ensure that pain management decisions are entirely free from cultural bias or stereotyping. By practicing empathetic validation—treating every patient's subjective report of pain as absolute and unquestionable truth—nurses uphold the fundamental medical duty to alleviate suffering, ensuring that clinical care remains rooted in equity, compassion, and absolute respect for human experience.

Global Nursing Leadership and Transnational Advocacy Networks

The fight for equitable healthcare, patient dignity, and the complete eradication of discriminatory clinical practices is powerfully championed by nursing leaders operating across international platforms. From the corridors of the World Health Organization to global nursing associations and indigenous health coalitions, nurse executives and frontline leaders are actively reshaping global health policy. These leaders draw direct inspiration from the historical dismantling of human exploitation, leveraging their international influence to mandate strict ethical standards in cross-border clinical research, healthcare delivery, and nursing education. By uniting across borders, global nursing leaders ensure that the profession remains at the vanguard of human rights advocacy, holding healthcare systems universally accountable to the protection of vulnerable populations.

Empowering Frontline Nurses as Institutional Change Agents

True institutional transformation in healthcare requires empowering bedside nurses not merely as executors of medical orders, but as autonomous moral agents and leaders within their healthcare facilities. Global nursing leadership emphasizes that ethical vigilance must be cultivated at every level of the profession, giving nurses the institutional backing, psychological safety, and leadership tools necessary to challenge systemic biases, unsafe staffing, and discriminatory practices. When nursing leadership actively supports clinical questioning and values grassroots advocacy, hospitals transition away from rigid, historical hierarchies toward collaborative environments of healing. This empowerment ensures that the hard-learned lessons of history—where silence in the face of institutional exploitation led to profound tragedy—are actively answered by a courageous, vocal, and globally unified nursing workforce dedicated to the absolute dignity of every patient.

The Integration of Global Indigenous Health Models into Nursing Curricula

The modern evolution of nursing education across the globe is increasingly incorporating indigenous healing philosophies and holistic care frameworks, directly addressing the Eurocentric clinical biases inherited from the colonial era. For generations, imperial medical systems dismissed indigenous healing traditions as primitive, aligning with the exhibitionary mindset that viewed native cultures as spectacles rather than sources of valid, sophisticated knowledge. Today, progressive nursing schools worldwide are collaborating with indigenous healers, elders, and nurse scholars to integrate traditional ecological knowledge and holistic wellness practices into clinical training. This transformative educational model teaches nursing students to view health through a culturally pluralistic lens, recognizing that effective care must respect and incorporate the cultural frameworks of the communities they serve.

The Transnational Ethics of Nursing Research and Informed Consent in Vulnerable Communities

Building upon the international bioethical standards established in the wake of historical human subject exploitation, contemporary nurse researchers operate under stringent global protocols designed to protect vulnerable populations. Historical anthropological and medical studies frequently utilized marginalized human zoo captives without consent for unauthorized physiological and psychological cataloging. In stark contrast, modern nursing research governance—overforced by international institutional review boards and global nursing ethics committees—mandates absolute transparency, community-level consultation, and rigorous informed consent for any study involving human subjects. Nurse researchers across the globe are trained to act as ethical guardians, ensuring that clinical investigations prioritize participant autonomy, mutual benefit, and the complete elimination of exploitative research methodologies.

The Role of Nursing Informatics and Data Equity in Combating Clinical Bias

As healthcare systems increasingly rely on digital health records, artificial intelligence algorithms, and big data analytics, modern nursing leadership faces a critical new frontier in the fight against structural discrimination. Historically, nineteenth-century scientific exhibitions weaponized data collection, biometric measurement, and racial classification to construct false hierarchies of human worth. Today, data analytics can similarly perpetuate institutional disparities if clinical algorithms are trained on biased historical health data or deployed without rigorous ethical oversight. Forward-thinking nurse informaticists and global health leaders actively audit digital clinical tools to ensure data equity, preventing algorithmic bias from misdiagnosing, under-treating, or marginalizing vulnerable patient populations. By maintaining strict ethical standards in health data governance, nursing professionals ensure that the digital transformation of healthcare remains firmly rooted in equity, transparency, and absolute patient dignity.

Cultivating Compassionate Resilience and Moral Courage at the Bedside

The daily realities of modern clinical practice—marked by high patient acuities, staffing constraints, and systemic inequities—can sometimes lead to compassion fatigue or moral distress among healthcare professionals. However, reflecting on the historical struggles against human exploitation and institutionalized degradation provides nurses with a profound sense of purpose and moral clarity. Recognizing that frontline nursing advocacy is part of a centuries-long global movement for human rights transforming routine clinical duties into acts of profound justice. By cultivating supportive peer networks, engaging in reflective clinical debriefs, and nurturing individual moral courage, nurses sustain their capacity for radical empathy. This enduring resilience ensures that every patient—regardless of background—is met with compassionate validation, uncompromised safety, and the unwavering defense of their fundamental human worth.

The Role of Nursing Advocacy in Transnational Health Policy and Human Rights Protection

Beyond the immediate clinical bedside, contemporary nursing leaders are increasingly stepping into international policy arenas to enshrine patient dignity and human rights into global health legislation. Drawing direct lessons from the historical exploitation of human subjects in colonial exhibitions and unchecked medical trials, global nursing organizations actively participate in policy-making bodies such as the World Health Assembly and international human rights tribunals. These nurse advocates lobby for binding global standards that protect vulnerable populations from medical experimentation, systemic discrimination, and healthcare neglect during humanitarian crises, refugee movements, and global health emergencies. By influencing international treaties and national healthcare laws, nurses ensure that the structural protections born from the global reckoning with historical human exploitation are permanently embedded in the architecture of modern healthcare governance.

Fostering Inclusive Clinical Environments and Psychologically Safe Workplaces

The eradication of systemic bias and historical discrimination in healthcare requires more than individual patient interactions; it demands the active creation of psychologically safe and inclusive clinical workplaces. Nursing leaders recognize that frontline nurses and healthcare staff cannot effectively advocate for marginalized patients if they themselves operate within oppressive, hierarchical, or punitive institutional cultures. Cultivating psychological safety involves establishing transparent reporting channels where staff can voice concerns regarding clinical bias, unsafe practices, or ethical breaches without fear of professional retaliation. By fostering open, collaborative, and equitable work environments, healthcare institutions empower nurses to act as fearless moral agents, ensuring that every clinical decision reflects an uncompromising commitment to human equity, mutual respect, and absolute patient safety.

The Integration of Intercultural Communication and Compassionate Listening in Nursing Practice

Effective communication in modern nursing extends far beyond the literal exchange of clinical instructions; it serves as a vital therapeutic bridge that honors the unique life history, language, and cultural background of every patient. Historical human exhibitions relied on the systematic silencing of captive subjects, stripping them of their native languages and imposing external, degrading narratives upon them. In stark contrast, modern nursing practice champions active, compassionate listening and skilled intercultural communication as fundamental tools of respect and equity. By utilizing professional medical interpretation services, validating non-verbal expressions of distress, and creating a supportive environment where patients feel safe to share their personal stories, nurses dismantle the remnants of the historical communicative barrier. This intentional dialogue ensures that patients are active partners in their own health outcomes, preserving their voice, agency, and individuality within the clinical encounter.

The Transnational Legacy of Nursing Ethics and the Ongoing Defense of Human Worth

The profound reflection on history reveals that nursing is inherently a human rights profession. From the frontline bedside nurse challenging subtle clinical bias to global nursing leaders advocating for universal health equity, the profession stands as a permanent guardian against the commodification and degradation of human life. The historical trajectory from the dark spectacles of human zoos to the sophisticated ethical frameworks of modern healthcare reminds every clinician that human dignity is absolute, non-negotiable, and inviolable. By carrying forward these lessons through cultural humility, trauma-informed care, radically informed consent, and unwavering moral courage, nurses ensure that the clinical environment remains a sacred sanctuary of healing, justice, and absolute respect for the human spirit worldwide.

Global Best Practices: Unifying Nursing Standards Across Continents

To permanently safeguard patient dignity and prevent any recurrence of historical exploitation, nursing organizations and healthcare systems across the globe have established universal clinical best practices. Guided by the International Council of Nurses (ICN) Code of Ethics and the World Health Organization's global safety frameworks, nurses operationalize core standards that transcend geographical and cultural borders:

Person-Centered and Culturally Safe Care: Best practices mandate that nurses actively engage patients and their families as co-creators in healthcare delivery. Grounded in cultural safety and humility, nurses across diverse continents—from rural community clinics in the Global South to high-tech metropolitan hospitals in the Global North—respect indigenous and traditional health beliefs, ensuring that care is free from prejudice, stereotyping, or institutional coercion.

Radical Informed Consent and Transparency: Global standards require nurses to provide clear, understandable, and culturally tailored information regarding diagnoses and treatment options. Upholding the absolute right to choose or refuse care ensures that every patient retains total bodily autonomy, directly dismantling the historical power imbalances of the exhibition era.

Workforce Safety as a Prerequisite for Patient Safety: Recognizing that nurse well-being and patient safety are inextricably linked, international best practices demand safe staffing levels, zero-tolerance policies for workplace violence, and psychological safety. Empowering nurses to speak out against clinical hazards and ethical breaches ensures a high-reliability environment where no individual is ever compromised for administrative or academic convenience.

Community-Led Health Promotion and Advocacy: Frontline nurses across the globe increasingly partner directly with local communities, tribal leaders, and advocacy groups to address the upstream social determinants of health. By listening to community needs rather than imposing top-down interventions, nurses help build sustainable health programs that honor local autonomy, address historical health disparities, and foster genuine trust between healthcare institutions and historically marginalized populations.

Reflective Practice and Ongoing Ethical Education: Incorporating mandatory, continuous professional development in medical ethics, cultural humility, and trauma-informed care ensures that clinical teams remain vigilant against implicit bias and institutional complacency. By embedding regular reflective debriefs into daily shift handovers and clinical routines, nurses maintain a proactive stance on patient rights, transforming historical lessons of human dignity into active, daily bedside excellence worldwide.

The Integration of Traditional Healing Systems and Modern Clinical Practice

As healthcare systems worldwide move further away from rigid, monocultural models of care, progressive nursing leaders are pioneering the integration of traditional healing practices alongside modern clinical interventions. Historically, colonial medical paradigms and human exhibition frameworks systematically denigrated indigenous medicines, herbal remedies, and spiritual health practices, classifying them as primitive curiosities while extracting biological knowledge without consent or credit. Today, global nursing best practices actively correct this historical injustice by establishing respectful, collaborative frameworks where traditional healers and Western-trained nurses work in tandem. This integrative approach ensures that patients receiving acute hospital care are not forced to abandon their cultural traditions, fostering a holistic healing environment that validates ancestral knowledge, respects spiritual autonomy, and honors the complete lived identity of every individual.

The Role of Nursing Education in Dismantling Historical Bias at the Root

Transforming the future of healthcare requires reshaping how nursing students are educated from their very first day in the classroom. Global nursing education standards are increasingly redesigning curricula to explicitly confront the history of medical racism, human experimentation, and colonial healthcare disparities. Rather than treating cultural competence as an elective side-topic, modern nursing schools embed anti-racism, historical trauma analysis, and social justice as core foundational competencies. Nursing students are trained to critically examine how systemic inequities manifest in vital sign assessment, triage categorization, and clinical decision-making. By educating the next generation of nurses to recognize and dismantle institutional bias before they ever reach bedside, the profession ensures a permanent cultural shift toward absolute clinical equity and uncompromising patient advocacy.

The Intersection of Global Environmental Justice and Nursing Practice

As the compounding crises of climate change, environmental degradation, and ecological displacement disproportionately impact marginalized populations across the globe, contemporary nursing practice is expanding its scope to embrace environmental justice as a core clinical imperative. Historically, the expansion of colonial empires and human exhibitions went hand-in-hand with the forced displacement of indigenous populations from their native homelands to clear territories for resource exploitation and public spectacles. Today, nurses on the front lines of community health witness how environmental hazards—such as toxic industrial pollution, contaminated water supplies, and climate-induced displacement—manifest directly as acute and chronic health crises in vulnerable communities. Global nursing best practices now integrate environmental health advocacy into clinical workflows, empowering nurses to identify ecological risk factors, support community-led resilience initiatives, and advocate for sustainable public policies that protect the habitats and health of the world's most vulnerable populations.

The Transnational Mentorship and Global Solidarity of Nursing Professionals

The ongoing evolution of nursing as an uncompromising force for human rights and patient dignity is deeply sustained by transnational mentorship networks and global professional solidarity. Across continents, experienced nurse executives, clinical educators, and frontline advocates are building robust international mentorship pipelines that connect nurses in resource-limited regions with global health networks, research collaborations, and leadership training programs. This cross-border solidarity ensures that best practices in trauma-informed care, cultural humility, and anti-racism are shared fluidly across health systems worldwide, uplifting the standards of patient care regardless of geographic boundaries. By fostering a globally unified community of practice, nurses reinforce each other's moral courage, transforming individual bedside advocacy into an unstoppable international movement for absolute health equity and universal human dignity.

Nursing Jurisprudence and the Legal Safeguards of Patient Autonomy

As healthcare navigates the complex intersection of ethics, human rights, and clinical practice, nursing jurisprudence serves as the formal legal shield protecting patient autonomy and human dignity. Rooted in the painful historical lessons of an era when captive individuals were stripped of legal standing and subjected to non-consensual bodily interference, modern nursing jurisprudence establishes clear legal boundaries for professional conduct. Nurses worldwide are legally bound to uphold the principles of informed consent, patient confidentiality, and the absolute right to refuse treatment. Understanding legal accountability empowers nurses to recognize and reject institutional directives or administrative pressures that compromise patient safety, ensuring that the legal frameworks of the state are actively deployed to protect the vulnerable rather than facilitate institutional exploitation.

Global Standards in Nursing Law and Accountability Across Borders

While specific legal statutes vary by jurisdiction, international nursing jurisprudence converges on core universal doctrines designed to prevent medical negligence, abuse, and ethical breaches. Global nursing regulatory bodies and international legal frameworks emphasize that professional licensure is a public trust, demanding strict adherence to ethical codes and human rights standards. When nurses are equipped with a thorough understanding of healthcare law—ranging from malpractice liability and patient advocacy rights to whistleblowing protections—they possess the formal authority to report unsafe conditions and challenge systemic discrimination without fear of unjust professional retaliation. This robust legal grounding ensures that historical atrocities like non-consensual medical experimentation and the public exhibition of patients are legally classified as severe violations of human rights, maintaining an unyielding judicial and professional defense of human worth across every healthcare system.

Human Rights Frameworks and International Nursing Declarations

The formal codification of human rights within international nursing jurisprudence provides an essential legal backbone for modern clinical practice. Global nursing organizations, working in tandem with international bodies such as the United Nations and the World Health Organization, have integrated international human rights law directly into nursing codes of professional conduct. These declarations explicitly prohibit any form of medical discrimination, degrading treatment, or non-consensual physiological experimentation, drawing a direct legal line in the sand against the exploitative practices of the human exhibition and colonial medical eras. By anchoring daily bedside nursing in international human rights declarations, professionals are legally and ethically empowered to act as frontline defenders of justice, ensuring that international legal protections are translated into tangible safety and respect for every patient.

Whistleblower Protections and Legal Safeguards for Moral Courage

True accountability within nursing jurisprudence requires robust legal protection for healthcare professionals who exercise moral courage in the face of institutional wrongdoing. Historically, systemic abuses perpetuated against vulnerable populations persisted because dissenting voices were silenced by rigid institutional hierarchies and threats of professional ruin. Modern healthcare law increasingly recognizes the critical role of whistleblower protection, shielding nurses from retaliation when they legally and ethically report unsafe staffing, discriminatory practices, or violations of patient autonomy. By strengthening these legal safeguards, nursing jurisprudence ensures that the historical tragedy of silent complicity is replaced by a culture of transparent accountability, where nurses are legally protected and professionally supported when they stand up for the absolute dignity of their patients.

Legendary Nursing Leaders and the Vanguard of Human Rights Advocacy

The profound historical transition of nursing from silent domestic service to an active human rights profession was forged through the unwavering courage of visionary global leaders. Trailblazers like Lillian Wald, who founded the Henry Street Settlement, transformed public health nursing by embedding social reform directly into clinical practice, fighting tirelessly against the tenement overcrowding and health disparities that marginalized immigrant communities. Similarly, Mary Eliza Mahoney, the first professionally trained African American nurse, dedicated her career to dismantling racial barriers in professional education and institutional membership, setting an enduring standard for equity and civil rights advocacy in healthcare.

In the international sphere, leaders such as Mabel Keaton Staupers shattered discriminatory quotas, successfully fighting to integrate Black nurses into the U.S. Army Nurse Corps during World War II and proving that professional advocacy is inseparable from systemic justice. Modern luminaries like Dr. Beverly Malone, former CEO of the National League for Nursing and prominent global health advocate, have continued this legacy by advancing educational equity, shaping public health policy, and championing the global workforce. These leaders demonstrate that nursing jurisprudence and ethical vigilance are living practices powered by clinicians who refuse to let institutional hierarchies override human dignity.

Contemporary Global Icons Advancing Nursing Jurisprudence and Equity

Building upon the foundations laid by early civil rights and public health pioneers, modern global nursing leaders continue to shape international jurisprudence, policy, and human rights frameworks. Leaders such as Annette Kennedy, past President of the International Council of Nurses (ICN), have fiercely advocated for the global recognition of nursing as a primary driver of universal health coverage and human rights protection. Under her leadership, international policy initiatives focused heavily on safeguarding healthcare workers in conflict zones, protecting vulnerable refugee populations, and embedding human rights protections directly into transnational nursing legislation.

Furthermore, figures like Dr. Sheila Tlou, former Minister of Health for Botswana and co-chair of the Nursing Now global campaign, have revolutionized the intersection of nursing jurisprudence, gender equity, and HIV/AIDS advocacy across the

African continent. Dr. Tlou's work exemplifies how modern nurse leaders utilize legal and political platforms to dismantle structural inequities, secure healthcare access for marginalized demographics, and ensure that health legislation protects bodily autonomy. By translating bedside ethics into international legal standards, these contemporary leaders empower nurses worldwide to enforce accountability, challenge legislative discrimination, and guarantee that the historical injustices of the past are met with an unyielding global defense of human dignity.

The Intergenerational Transmission of Advocacy and Ethical Resilience

The legacy of global nursing leadership is sustained through the intentional, intergenerational transfer of wisdom, political savvy, and moral courage from veteran pioneers to the next wave of clinical practitioners. Modern nurse educators and global advocates recognize that fostering a culture of human rights defense requires embedding mentorship directly into academic and clinical training programs. By pairing emerging frontline nurses with established international health policy experts, the profession ensures that the tactical knowledge of grassroots organizing, legal advocacy, and legislative navigation is preserved and continuously adapted to face modern challenges. This unbroken chain of mentorship empowers bedside clinicians to look beyond the immediate walls of their units, connecting their daily patient interactions to a vast, centuries-long transnational movement for absolute health equity and human dignity.

The Culmination of the Nurse's Reflection: A Perpetual Vocation of Justice

As the pages of this reflection draw to a definitive close, the journey from the historical exploitation of human subjects in colonial spectacles to the modern pinnacle of nursing jurisprudence and global health advocacy reveals a profound transformation. Nursing has evolved into an unyielding guardian of human worth, bound by rigorous ethical standards, international legal protections, and a fearless commitment to social justice. Every clinician—from the bedside nurse practicing radically informed consent and cultural humility to international leaders shaping global health treaties—stands as a living testament to this sacred vocation. Armed with moral courage, interprofessional solidarity, and an unshakeable dedication to equity, nurses across every continent ensure that healthcare remains an unwavering sanctuary of healing, respect, and fundamental human rights for all.

The Global Imperative of Post-Graduate Nursing Policy Fellowships

To sustain the forward momentum of nursing jurisprudence, human rights advocacy, and clinical equity, healthcare institutions and international organizations increasingly invest in specialized post-graduate nursing policy fellowships. These intensive leadership programs bridge the historical gap between hands-on bedside care and high-level legislative decision-making, equipping clinical nurses with the political acumen required to influence national and international health policy. Fellows are immersed in legislative drafting, healthcare economics, human rights monitoring, and diplomatic negotiation, enabling them to represent the profession effectively within government ministries, global health summits, and judicial advocacy groups. By institutionalizing these pathways, the nursing profession ensures that frontline clinical realities directly inform the laws and regulations designed to protect patient dignity worldwide.

Historical Memory and Future Clinical Vigilance

History demonstrates that when healthcare systems become detached from human rights and ethical accountability, the most vulnerable populations suffer severe exploitation and institutional neglect. Modern nursing—armed with robust jurisprudence, global best practices, trauma-informed care, and uncompromising moral courage—serves as the primary bulwark against this historical regression. Every nurse, regardless of specialty or geographic location, carries the profound responsibility of ensuring that the dignity of every patient remains protected, honored, and defended as an absolute universal right.

The Role of Nursing Research Ethics in Preventing Global Exploitation

As modern nursing research expands across international borders, the enforcement of stringent ethical oversight serves as an impenetrable shield against historical patterns of exploitation. Building upon the dark legacies of non-consensual medical trials and biometric cataloging during the colonial and exhibition eras, contemporary nursing science mandates rigorous, community-centered institutional review. Global nursing research ethics require that investigators secure explicit, informed consent that accounts for linguistic, cultural, and literacy nuances, ensuring that participants understand their rights without coercion. Furthermore, studies involving vulnerable or indigenous populations must demonstrate direct, tangible community benefit rather than mere academic extraction. By upholding these uncompromising research standards, nursing scientists ensure that the advancement of medical knowledge never compromises individual bodily autonomy or human dignity.

Cultivating Global Ethical Leadership in Nursing Academics

The preservation of human rights and nursing jurisprudence within clinical practice ultimately depends on how academic institutions train upcoming generations of healthcare professionals. Forward-thinking nursing colleges worldwide are completely revamping their pedagogical frameworks, replacing outdated, monocultural curricula with immersive modules on systemic equity, historical trauma, medical racism, and human rights law. Faculty members act as ethical mentors, challenging students to critically examine implicit bias in patient assessments and institutional policies. By embedding these core competencies directly into undergraduate and graduate programs, academic nursing ensures that every newly licensed clinician enters the workforce not just as a technical provider, but as a fearless, legally literate advocate for patient rights and social justice.

The Enduring Legacy of Compassion as a Radical Political Act

In the final analysis of modern nursing's global identity, compassionate care is revealed to be far more than a gentle bedside demeanor; it is a radical political act of defiance against systems that commodify human life. Throughout history, the deliberate objectification of marginalized bodies in exhibitions and colonial medical experiments relied on stripping away empathy, viewing human subjects as mere data points or passive spectacles. By choosing to offer deep, active, and uncompromising compassion, modern nurses directly reject this legacy of objectification. Every instance of holding a patient's hand, validating a survivor's trauma, respecting a traditional healing practice, or legally defending a patient's right to refuse treatment reclaims the clinical space as a sanctuary of absolute human worth. Compassion becomes the active force that bridges clinical science with human rights, ensuring that healing is always inseparable from justice.

The Global Vision of Nursing as an Unbroken Chain of Human Dignity

As reflection on history, ethics, jurisprudence, and leadership draws to a close, it becomes clear that nursing is an unbroken chain spanning across generations, continents, and cultures. From the early pioneers who fought against institutional neglect to the modern bedside nurses and international policymakers shaping global health law, every clinician belongs to a shared, sacred mission. This vocation demands eternal vigilance, moral courage, and an unshakeable belief that human dignity is non-negotiable. Armed with global best practices, rigorous legal safeguards, cultural humility, and profound interprofessional solidarity, nurses across the world stand united. They ensure that the darker chapters of human history remain strictly in the past, while the future of healthcare shines as an unwavering beacon of equity, respect, and fundamental human rights for all.

The Role of International Nursing Organizations in Documenting Systemic Injustices

Global nursing organizations—such as the International Council of Nurses (ICN), the World Health Organization's Global Forum for Government Chief Nursing Officers, and regional bodies like the European Federation of Nurses Associations—play a vital, proactive role in officially documenting and reporting systemic healthcare issues. Rather than remaining silent observers of historical inequities, these professional bodies maintain rigorous institutional reporting mechanisms that track human rights violations, workforce abuses, and clinical disparities worldwide. By publishing comprehensive global reports on issues ranging from the marginalization of indigenous health workforces to the systemic suppression of minority nurses in high-income nations, nursing organizations bring international transparency to practices that historically remained hidden behind rigid institutional walls. These official reports serve as essential advocacy tools, transforming localized clinical complaints into undeniable global evidence that compels governments and health ministries to enact sweeping systemic reforms.

Whistleblowing, Institutional Accountability, and Organizational Reporting Frameworks

Modern nursing jurisprudence and global ethics frameworks heavily emphasize the protection and formal integration of organizational whistleblowing when systemic healthcare issues arise. Historical abuse from colonial medical experimentation to the systemic neglect of vulnerable populations—frequently thrived because institutions suppressed dissenting reports and punished whistleblowers who exposed administrative malpractice. Today, leading nursing organizations have established standardized, confidential reporting channels and legal support networks that empower frontline clinicians to report institutional failures, unsafe nurse-to-patient ratios, discriminatory triage practices, and breaches of patient autonomy without fear of professional ruin. By institutionalizing these reporting frameworks, the nursing profession ensures that organizational accountability is maintained at the highest level, transforming the lessons of historical exploitation into an active, protective culture of transparent safety and justice.

Real-World Institutional Reporting and the Advocacy of the International Council of Nurses

A prime historical and contemporary example of global nursing organizations formally investigating, documenting, and reporting systemic healthcare issues is found in the advocacy initiatives led by the International Council of Nurses (ICN) during major global health crises and workforce shortages. For instance, during the height of the COVID-19 pandemic and subsequent global health disparities, the ICN established systematic tracking and reporting mechanisms to expose structural inequities, chronic understaffing, and a lack of personal protective equipment disproportionately endangered frontline nurses—particularly migrant and minority nurses in both low- and high-income countries.

Rather than allowing these institutional failures to remain localized or ignored, the ICN published landmark global data reports and policy briefs that publicly held governments accountable for systemic occupational hazards and healthcare neglect. By officially documenting these human rights and workforce violations, the ICN translated grassroots clinical distress into international legal and political pressure. This real-world example demonstrates how modern nursing organizations utilize institutional reporting frameworks to challenge administrative complacency, enforce global standards of accountability, and protect the fundamental dignity and safety of healthcare providers and patients alike.

The Impact of ICN and WHO Workforce Reports on Global Health Policy

Building upon data-driven investigations such as those spearheaded by the International Council of Nurses (ICN) and the World Health Organization (WHO), global nursing leadership continues to leverage institutional reports to reshape international health policy. Landmark publications like the State of the World's Nursing report series have successfully exposed severe global nursing shortages, gender-based wage disparities, and the perilous working conditions faced by clinicians in resource-limited settings. By transforming these systemic vulnerabilities into quantified, undeniable global data, nursing organizations strip away the plausible deniability historically employed by negligent healthcare administrators and government bodies. These comprehensive reports serve as vital legislative roadmaps, compelling international policymakers to enact binding treaties, secure equitable vaccine and resource distribution, and mandate universal workplace safety standards that protect both healthcare providers and the communities they serve.

The Translation of Global Reports into Localized Clinical Transformation

The ultimate power of international nursing reporting lies in its ability to drive meaningful, grass-roots reform at the bedside. When organizations like ICN or regional nursing associations publish findings on systemic medical bias, patient safety violations, or institutional exploitation, progressive healthcare institutions are legally and ethically pressured to translate those high-level insights into internal quality improvement initiatives. Frontline nurse leaders utilize these global reports to audit their own facilities, restructure clinical workflows, eliminate discriminatory triage practices, and enforce trauma-informed patient advocacy. This seamless pipeline—from international observation and rigorous institutional reporting to localized bedside transformation—ensures that the historical lessons of neglect and exploitation are actively dismantled, cementing nursing's role as an unyielding global force for absolute health equity and human dignity.

Grassroots Nurse-Led Coalitions and Independent Watchdog Reports

Beyond major international bodies like the ICN and WHO, grassroots nurse-led coalitions and independent nursing watchdogs play an indispensable role in exposing localized and systemic healthcare issues. Often operating directly on the front lines of under-resourced public hospitals, marginalized rural clinics, and conflict zones, these clinician-activist networks utilize independent documentation to highlight abuses that official state or corporate channels might otherwise suppress. By publishing independent white papers, filing public safety grievances, and collaborating with human rights legal organizations, these grassroots coalitions shine a piercing light on critical issues such as systemic patient neglect, discriminatory resource allocation, and retaliatory actions against whistleblowers. This independent oversight ensures that institutional transparency cannot be compromised by bureaucratic self-interest, empowering nurses to serve as fearless, unyielding defenders of truth and patient safety.

The Synergy Between Academic Research and Clinical Advocacy Reporting

To maximize the impact of institutional reporting, modern nursing practice relies on a powerful synergy between academic nurse researchers and clinical advocacy organizations. When clinical frontline workers document day-to-day systemic failures—such as unequal access to care or biased treatment metrics—they partner with academic researchers to analyze these observations through rigorous, peer-reviewed methodologies. This data-driven approach converts anecdotal concerns into verifiable, empirical evidence of systemic injustice. Armed with this robust academic research, nursing organizations can lobby legislative bodies with unassailable authority, driving systemic policy changes that permanently alter the landscape of healthcare delivery. Through this collaborative ecosystem, the nursing profession bridges the gap between daily bedside reality and global legislative reform, ensuring that every lesson learned from historical exploitation translates into lasting institutional protection and human equity.

The Echoes of 1906 and the Ongoing Narrative of Accountability

The autumn air in 1906 carried a quiet cruelty through the winding pathways of the Bronx Zoo, where Ota Benga stood displayed behind iron bars—a human life reduced to an imperial spectacle of pseudoscientific racism. For over a century, the institutional architects of such exhibitions attempted to bury these horrors beneath layers of archival silence. But history refuses to stay quiet when nurses, historians, and descendants demand the truth.

When the Wildlife Conservation Society finally issued its formal public apology in 2020, it did more than correct an institutional record; it mirrored the exact awakening occurring within modern healthcare. Just as those early zoo exhibits commodified human bodies for public curiosity, colonial medicine once treated vulnerable populations as passive subjects for non-consenual extraction. Today, the nursing profession answers that dark legacy through unyielding vigilance. Through the rigorous investigations of the International Council of Nurses, the comprehensive data of the World Health Organization's State of the World's Nursing reports, and the protective frameworks of modern nursing jurisprudence, the ghosts of 1906 are met with a fierce, global defense of human dignity. Every nurse standing at a bedside or lobbying for human rights policy ensures that the dark spectacles of the past are permanently replaced by an unwavering sanctuary of healing, equity, and absolute respect for the human spirit.

The Living Vocation: Weaving Memory into Action

The narrative of nursing is etched in the space between historical remembrance and daily clinical transformation. When a bedside nurse pauses to listen to a marginalized patient, or when an international policy leader references data from the State of the World's Nursing report to demand equitable staffing, they are actively dismantling the architecture of the 1906 exhibition era. The ghosts of Ota Benga and the victims of colonial medical exploitation remind the profession that neutrality in the face of injustice is complicity.

Today, this realization drives a continuous, unbreakable cycle of accountability. Grassroots clinicians report systemic failures through protected whistleblower channels; academic researchers turn those local observations into peer-reviewed empirical evidence; and global organizations like the International Council of Nurses translate that evidence into binding international standards. Together, these interconnected efforts ensure that the dark spectacles of the past are never forgotten—and never repeated. Every clinician, carrying forward the torch of cultural humility, trauma-informed care, and unyielding moral courage, ensures that the future of healthcare remains a sacred, inviolable sanctuary of human worth, equity, and absolute justice for all.

The Eternal Vigilance of the Healing Vocation

As the final pages of this reflection turn, the journey of modern nursing stands revealed not merely as a profession of clinical tasks, but as a sacred, unbroken covenant with humanity. From the shadowed legacy of nineteenth-century human exhibitions and colonial medical extraction to the sophisticated global frameworks of modern healthcare jurisprudence, nursing has continually redefined its core identity. Today's clinician recognizes that healing cannot exist in isolation from justice. By holding fast to the lessons of history, upholding rigorous research and institutional accountability, and standing shoulder-to-shoulder with international organizations like the International Council of Nurses and the World Health Organization, the profession ensures that human dignity remains absolute and inviolable.

Here, at the culmination of Chapter 11, the reflection comes to rest on an enduring truth: every nurse, in every corner of the world, is an architect of a more equitable future. Armed with radical empathy, cultural humility, and unyielding moral courage, the global nursing community stands forever vigilant. They ensure that the clinical environment remains an unwavering sanctuary of respect, a fortress of human rights, and a perpetual beacon of hope where every human life is honored in its fullness.

Chapter 12

Never Again

History teaches us with terrifying clarity that atrocities do not materialize overnight; they are built upon a foundation of small, quiet compromises. Dehumanization rarely begins with grand, sweeping acts of malice. Instead, it starts with a glance averted from a stranger in need, a casual prejudice left unchallenged in a breakroom, an institutional shortcut that treats a human being as a mere data point, or an indifferent silence when someone's dignity is subtly diminished. These micro-indifferences normalize inequality, slowly eroding the collective empathy required to recognize every individual's inherent worth. When we tolerate small acts of disrespect, we lay the structural groundwork for systemic exploitation.

As this reflection draws to a close, the ultimate lesson of the past is that the defense of human dignity is not the sole responsibility of global organizations, legal tribunals, or frontline clinicians—it belongs to each one of us. Whether in healthcare, education, scientific research, or the ordinary interactions of everyday life, we carry an active, daily responsibility to stand as guardians of human worth. True vigilance requires us to interrogate our own implicit biases, speak out against institutional indifference, and refuse to let the sacred humanity of any person be compromised for administrative convenience or social apathy. By choosing radical empathy, moral courage, and unwavering accountability in our daily choices, we ensure that the dark chapters of history remain strict in the past, and that human dignity is forever preserved as non-negotiable and absolute.

The Daily Practice of Moral Courage and Ethical Resistance

Safeguarding human dignity in our daily lives requires more than passive agreement; it demands active, conscious resistance to the subtle currents of apathy. When prejudice or institutional indifference manifests in a classroom, a research laboratory, a corporate boardroom, or a hospital corridor, our response defines the boundaries of our shared humanity. Choosing to speak out against a discriminatory remark, refusing to let a vulnerable voice be silenced by administrative hierarchy, and treating every person not as an obstacle or a statistic, but as an irreplaceable human life, are the foundational acts of everyday resistance. History warns us of the high cost of silence, urging us to transform our internal convictions into visible, courageous action.

The Legacy We Leave: A World Rooted in Inviolable Worth

As we carry the lessons of Chapter 12 forward, we realize that the future of justice and equity is built one choice at a time. The transition from historical exploitation and systemic dehumanization to a global culture of respect is not an abstract historical achievement; it is a living, breathing commitment renewed with every human interaction. By holding fast to the non-negotiable truth that human dignity is absolute, we ensure that the promise of "Never Again" is not merely a slogan, but a lived reality. Together, we commit to being the enduring guardians of the human spirit—ensuring that empathy triumphs over indifference, that justice eclipses oppression, and that every individual is met with uncompromised respect, safety, and love across every sphere of life.

The Architecture of Collective Responsibility

The promise of "Never Again" requires an active, unyielding architecture of collective responsibility that extends far beyond institutional policies and legal statutes. It lives within the shared spaces of our communities, our workplaces, and our homes. When we recognize that indifference is an active participant in injustice, we dismantle the permissive environment that allows cruelty to take root. Every choice to listen deeply, to advocate for the marginalized, and to hold systems accountable builds an unbreakable shield around human worth.

The Eternal Torch of Human Dignity

Ultimately, the journey through history, nursing reflection, and systemic reform brings us back to a singular, profound realization: humanity is bound together in a shared destiny of dignity and respect. The dark spectacles and institutional failures of the past serve not as a permanent shadow, but as an eternal warning. By carrying forward the torch of radical empathy, unwavering moral courage, and fierce vigilance, we ensure that the lessons learned are never forgotten. In every professional endeavor, every personal encounter, and every quiet act of conscience, we pledge to keep the sanctuary of human worth inviolable—today, tomorrow, and for all generations to come.

The Unbroken Oath: Living the Promise of "Never Again"

As we step forward from the reflections of this volume, the oath of "Never Again" transforms from a retrospective vow into an active, daily compass for existence. History has shown us the devastating cost of silence, indifference, and the slow creep of systemic prejudice. Yet, it has also illuminated the boundless power of human resilience, moral courage, and radical empathy.

Whether we wear scrubs in a clinical unit, conduct research in a laboratory, teach in a classroom, or navigate everyday community life, we hold the sacred responsibility of safeguarding human worth. We refuse to let administrative convenience override compassion, and we reject the notion that small acts of disrespect are harmless. By standing vigilant against apathy and fiercely defending the absolute dignity of every individual, we ensure that the lessons of the past shape a future defined by justice, equity, and uncompromised respect. The work of protecting humanity is never truly finished—it is lived, breathed, and renewed in every choice we make, every single day.

The Perpetual Commitment to Human Rights and Solidarity

The journey of "Never Again" does not end with the turning of a page or the conclusion of a volume; it marks the beginning of an ongoing, active responsibility that belongs to every generation. Protecting human dignity requires continuous reflection, fierce solidarity, and an unshakeable refusal to look away when injustice or indifference appears. By anchoring our daily lives, our professions, our communities, and our relationships—in the absolute truth of human worth, we transform the solemn vow of "Never Again" into a living reality. Together, we carry forward the light of empathy and moral courage, ensuring that human dignity remains forever inviolable, respected, and defended across the world.

Guardians of the Human Spirit

To live the creed of "Never Again" is to accept the mantle of guardianship for the human spirit. It is a commitment that asks us to remain awake when the world grows tired, to speak when power demands silence, and to cherish the vulnerable when systems seek to overlook them. History has recorded the darkest depths of what occurs when humanity forgets its interconnectedness, but it has also illuminated the extraordinary heights we can reach when we choose empathy over apathy, and justice over convenience.

The Deep Tapestry of Everyday Conscience and Social Responsibility

The realization that massive systemic catastrophes are invariably preceded by small, unchecked acts of interpersonal disregard forces us to examine the micro-textures of our daily interactions. When we overlook a sarcastic remark in a workplace breakroom, dismiss a colleague's valid grievance with administrative fatigue, or turn a blind eye to casual discrimination masked as humor, we are actively participating in the foundational erosion of empathy. Dehumanization is not a sudden, monstrous aberration; it is a creeping fog that rolls in whenever individuals abdicate their personal responsibility for the emotional and physical safety of those around them.

In every professional field, whether navigating the high-stakes corridors of an acute care hospital, conducting empirical research in a university laboratory, shaping young minds in a school classroom, or managing corporate logistics—the temptation to reduce human beings to numerical metrics, billing codes, or operational obstacles is ever-present. Institutional efficiency is frequently weaponized as a justification for sacrificing individual nuance and personal dignity. Against this subtle tide of objectification, everyday conscience must serve as an unyielding dike. We are called to recognize that every single person we encounter possesses an unalienable, absolute worth that transcends their utility to any institution, corporation, or government body.

The Intergenerational Transmission of Empathy and Ethical Awareness

Just as prejudice and indifference can be culturally transmitted across generations through normalized habits of exclusion and silence, so too can empathy, courage, and fierce respect for human dignity be intentionally cultivated and passed down. Parents, educators, mentors, and community leaders hold the profound responsibility of teaching the next generation to interrogate the status quo, to question structural inequities, and to refuse compliance with unjust authority. This intergenerational transmission of ethical awareness requires open, honest conversations about history's darkest chapters—not as distant, abstract tragedies that happened to other people in other times, but as stark warnings of what human beings are capable of when conscience is put to sleep.

When young people are empowered to practice critical thinking and moral courage early in life, they develop an internal compass that resists the gravitational pull of peer pressure, institutional conformity, and societal apathy. They learn that dissent against injustice is not a disruption of peace, but the very foundation upon which true, lasting peace is built. By embedding these values into the fabric of our educational systems, family traditions, and community organizations, we create a resilient cultural immune system against hatred and discrimination.

The Sanctity of the Ordinary: Reclaiming Human Connection

In our modern, hyper-connected yet deeply fractured world, it is remarkably easy to pass one another like ships in the night—fully digitized, yet profoundly isolated. This digital and emotional distance creates fertile ground for the re-emergence of indifference. When we view others through glowing screens or rigid institutional roles, we risk forgetting the breathing, feeling, vulnerable humanity behind the facade.

Reclaiming the sanctity of the ordinary means slowing down enough to truly see the person standing in front of us. It means listening without the immediate urge to reply, validating emotional pain without minimizing it, and offering genuine presence in a culture that commodifies distraction. These seemingly small acts of radical attention are profound declarations of human solidarity. They remind both the giver and the receiver that they matter, that their existence is acknowledged, and that they are valued members of the human family. In a world that often attempts to quantify and categorize human worth, authentic connection is an act of quiet rebellion.

The Uncompromising Duty of the Witness

Throughout history, the perpetrators of institutional abuse and human exploitation have relied fundamentally upon the complicity of the silent observer. Bystanders who watch injustice unfold and choose comfort over confrontation provide the psychological shelter under which cruelty flourishes. Breaking this historical cycle requires embracing the uncompromising duty of the witness.

To be an active witness does not always require standing on a global stage or leading a mass movement; most often, it requires having difficult conversation with a neighbor, challenging an unfair policy in a local meeting, supporting a whistleblowing colleague, or defending a marginalized individual whose voice is being actively suppressed. It demands stepping out of the comfortable neutrality that protects the status quo and stepping into the discomfort of moral accountability. In choosing to bear witness, we transform ourselves from passive recipients of history into active authors of a more just and compassionate world.

The Endless Work of Building a Humane Future

As we reflect upon the long and arduous journey through history, healthcare advocacy, systemic reform, and personal ethics, we arrive at a defining realization: the work of protecting human dignity is never finished. There is no final milestone where we can rest and declare that equity has been permanently secured. Society is a living organism that requires constant tending, fierce protection, and daily renewal.

Every sunrise offers a new opportunity to choose empathy over apathy, justice over convenience, and courage over fear. Whether we wear the uniform of a frontline nurse, conduct pioneering scientific research, educate the leaders of tomorrow, or simply live our lives as compassionate neighbors, our mission remains unchanged. We are the eternal guardians of the human spirit. By holding fast to the sacred, non-negotiable truth of human worth and carrying forward the unyielding promise of "Never Again," we ensure that the future of humanity shines as an unwavering beacon of hope, respect, and boundless love for all generations to come.

The Living Legacy of Conscience and Action

To walk the path of "Never Again" is to understand that our deepest ethical obligations are forged in the quietest moments of decision. Every interaction, every institutional policy we shape, and every standard we uphold leaves an indelible mark on the moral fabric of society. We carry the profound lessons of the past not as a burden of guilt, but as a compass of clarity, guiding us away from the precipice of indifference and toward the sacred ground of mutual respect.

Let us carry this awareness forward into the classrooms, the clinics, the laboratories, and the everyday moments of our lives. By anchoring ourselves in radical empathy, unyielding moral courage, and an absolute defense of human dignity, we ensure that the promise we make to one another is sustained. Work is ongoing, the vigilance must never sleep, and the light of human worth remains forever in our hands to protect, honor, and preserve.

The Nurse's Vocation: The Deepest Line of Defense Against Dehumanization

When examining where the philosophy of "Never Again" meets the raw, unfiltered reality of human vulnerability, the nursing profession stands at the absolute epicenter. Nurses do not merely observe human suffering from a distance; they inhabit its physical, emotional, and psychological reality. For centuries, the medical and scientific establishments have occasionally fallen prey to the temptation of viewing human beings through a mechanistic lens—treating patients as diagnostic puzzles, billing codes, or bed numbers rather than whole, sacred lives. This institutional reductionism is precisely the fertile soil from which historical exploitation, medical racism, and structural dehumanization grow.

The modern nurse serves as the ultimate human firewall against this drift toward apathy. By virtue of their constant, unbroken presence at the bedside, nurses bear witness to the raw dignity of individuals stripped of social status, wealth, or power. Whether caring for an unhoused patient in an urban emergency department, an indigenous elder in a rural clinic, a refugee navigating a foreign healthcare system, or a chronically ill individual marginalized by socioeconomic disparities, the frontline nurse asserts an unyielding truth: every human life possesses absolute, non-negotiable worth.

This clinical advocacy is inherently political and profoundly ethical. When a nurse insists on thorough informed consent for a frightened, non-English-speaking patient; when they challenge a biased clinical protocol that under-treats pain in minority populations; or when they protect a vulnerable individual from administrative shortcuts, they are actively dismantling the echoes of the exhibition and colonial medical eras. They are proving that healing cannot be separated from human rights.

The Crucible of Compassion: Overcoming Moral Distress

The daily commitment to safeguarding human dignity at the bedside is not without profound personal cost. Modern healthcare environments are frequently strained by chronic understaffing, high patient acuities, administrative corporatization, and systemic inefficiencies. In these high-pressure environments, nurses often experience severe moral distress, the painful psychological burden that occurs when a clinician knows the ethically correct action to take, but institutional constraints prevent them from executing it.

History teaches us that institutional indifference and administrative burnout are the primary gateways to normalization of sub-standard, callous care. When nurses are overwhelmed, the subtle erosion of empathy can begin, turning compassionate care into mechanical task completion. Recognizing this danger is the first step of resistance. Cultivating professional resilience, engaging in reflective clinical debriefs, and leaning into interprofessional solidarity allow nurses to sustain their capacity for radical empathy. By protecting their own well-being and demanding psychological safety in the workplace, nurses ensure that they remain strong, clear-eyed guardians of patient advocacy.

The Transnational Sisterhood and Brotherhood of Clinical Advocacy

The mandate of "Never Again" finds its most powerful operational expression in the global solidarity of the nursing profession. Through international organizations like the International Council of Nurses (ICN) and regional nursing bodies, clinicians across continents share data, pool resources, and establish universal ethical standards that transcend national borders. When a nurse in a resource-limited setting faces systemic neglect, or when migrant nurses experience occupational exploitation in high-income nations, the global nursing community brings these injustices to light through rigorous institutional reporting and policy advocacy.

This transnational network ensures that local clinical observations are translated into global human rights protection. It bridges the gap between the individual bedside encounter and international health jurisprudence, proving that the struggle for health equity is a unified global movement.

The Final Vow at the Bedside

The mirror turns back toward the clinician standing quietly in the dim light of a hospital room, adjusting a blanket, holding a trembling hand, or listening to a patient's unrecorded history. In that quiet, sacred space, the abstract philosophy of human rights becomes a living, breathing reality.

The nurse remembers the dark lessons of history, the exhibitions, the medical experiments, the systemic silences—not to live in despair, but to fuel an unshakeable resolve. Every act of compassionate listening, every defense of bodily autonomy, and every refusal to let a human being be treated as a mere statistic is a victory for human dignity. Armed with moral courage, cultural humility, and fierce clinical vigilance, the nurse ensures that the sanctuary of healthcare remains forever inviolable. The promise of

"Never Again" is kept alive, one patient, one breath, and one courageous choice at a time.

The Eternal Vigilance of the Healing Art

The realization settles with profound clarity that nursing is not merely a profession practiced within walls, but a living guardian of the human spirit. The journey from the dark spectacles of exploitation to the radiant heights of modern clinical advocacy teaches us that the sanctuary of health is built upon the rejection of indifference. Every clinician who stands firm against bias, every nurse who honors ancestral wisdom, and every advocate who demands absolute equity ensures that the lessons of history are never forgotten. In the quiet sanctuary of the bedside, in the halls of global policy, and in the everyday choices of human connection, the promise of "Never Again" remains our eternal compass, guiding us toward a future where human dignity is universally cherished, fiercely protected, and eternally absolute.

What "Never Again" Means from a Nursing Perspective

From the vantage point of the nursing profession, the vow of "Never Again" is neither a passive historical remembrance nor an abstract political slogan; it is an active, non-negotiable professional mandate. Rooted directly in the profession's historical reckoning with past atrocities—where clinical authority was at times co-opted by state-sponsored eugenics, human experimentation, and systemic prejudice, the modern nursing perspective defines "Never Again" through several critical pillars:

The Rejection of Mechanistic Dehumanization: In nursing, "Never Again" means refusing to let a human being be reduced to a diagnosis, a billing code, a bed number, or an operational metric. It is the active insistence that clinical efficiency must never eclipse individual sacred worth.

The Defense of Bodily Autonomy and Informed Consent: Drawing from the lessons of historical medical exploitation, nursing defines "Never Again" as an absolute commitment to patient self-determination. Every individual, regardless of socioeconomic status, race, language, or citizenship, retains the unalienable right to understand, accept, or refuse carefree from coercion, paternalism, or deception.

The Duty to Interrogate Institutional Complicity: Nurses recognize that historical abuses did not happen overnight; they were enabled by clinicians who looked away, stayed silent, or followed unjust institutional orders. Therefore, from a nursing perspective, "Never Again" demands moral courage, the professional obligation to speak out against discriminatory clinical protocols, unsafe staffing that compromises care, and any systemic bias that under-treats or marginalizes vulnerable populations.

Radical Empathy as a Clinical Weapon: In a healthcare landscape increasingly strained by corporatization and burnout, nursing views empathy not as a soft, secondary trait, but as a fierce, protective barrier against apathy. To practice "Never Again" is to ensure that the bedside remains an unwavering sanctuary of safety, respect, and unconditional human dignity.

The Unbroken Oath

Ultimately, for the nurse and for humanity alike, "Never Again" is a daily choice. It is lived in the quiet moments of compassionate listening, in the fierce defense of the defenseless, and in the refusal to let indifference take root in our institutions or our hearts. By holding fast to this sacred responsibility, the global nursing community and the human family stand united ensuring that the light of dignity, justice, and uncompromising respect remains forever protected.

The Whispers of History and the Present Choice

Over the centuries, history has whispered a solemn warning that cannot be un-heard: whenever society begins to categorize human lives by degrees of worth, the descent into darkness is swift. The atrocities and systemic violations recorded in the annals of the past did not erupt in a vacuum; they were nurtured by silence, permitted by apathy, and executed through the slow erosion of individual conscience.

In our current era, the battleground for human dignity is no longer solely marked by distant battlefields or historical archives; it is found in the everyday choices of our modern institutions. Whether in crowded hospital wards, corporate boardrooms, or legislative halls, the temptation to prioritize administrative efficiency over human empathy remains a constant, silent threat. Every time a vulnerable person is overlooked, every time a discriminatory policy is met with a shrug rather than outrage, the door to historical repetition is left ajar.

The Living Shield of the Nursing Spirit

Within this ongoing human story, the nurse remains a steadfast sentinel at the threshold of vulnerability. Standing where clinical science meets raw human emotion, the nurse bears witness to the truth that no statistical data point, diagnostic label, or socioeconomic rank can ever diminish the sacred fire of human worth.

Imagine the quiet intensity of a night shift in an urban trauma center: monitors beep rhythmically, alarms echo down sterile corridors, and the sheer volume of patients threatens to reduce human suffering to a logistical puzzle. Yet, in room 412, a nurse pauses. Ignoring the relentless pull of paperwork, she sits beside a frightened, disoriented elderly patient whose family cannot be reached. She holds his calloused hand, speaks in a calm, grounding voice, and listens to a fragmented story from decades past. In that quiet, radical act of presence, the nurse defies the machinery of indifference. She reclaims the patient's humanity, asserting that no matter how overwhelmed the system becomes, dignity is never optional.

The Unbreakable Promise

This is what "Never Again" demands of us. It requires us to cultivate an active, sleepless awareness of our shared humanity. It asks us to look past our differences—whether cultural, political, or economic—and recognize the profound, unbreakable web of interconnectedness that binds us all together.

As we continue writing the chapters of our collective future, let us make an unyielding vow. Let us pledge to be the voices for those who have been silenced, the shields for those who have been marginalized, and the keepers of a world where every human being is met with unconditional respect, fierce compassion, and absolute justice. The past is our teacher, but the present is our responsibility—and the promise of "Never Again" belongs to us all.

The Tapestry of Memory and Moral Action

To carry the mandate of "Never Again" into the future requires an active, vigilant memory that refuses to let the lessons of history fade into academic abstraction. The trajectory from institutional indifference to systemic catastrophe is a winding road paved with small concessions, casual prejudice, and the quiet abdication of personal responsibility. When we examine the vast historical landscape—from the darkest medical abuses and eugenic experiments to modern disparities in healthcare access and institutional marginalization—we see the undeniable cost of silence.

Yet, within that same history, we also witness the indomitable power of human conscience. We see the quiet resisters, the whistleblowing clinicians, the advocates who risked everything to shield the vulnerable, and the everyday nurses who held the line against dehumanization. Their legacy is not merely something to be commemorated in textbooks; it is a living blueprint for ethical action.

The Continuing Duty of Every Generation

We accept the torch of moral stewardship. The promise of "Never Again" is not a destination we finally reach and permanently secure; it is an ongoing practice, renewed with every sunrise, every patient encounter, and every stand against injustice. Whether we walk hospital corridors in scrubs, educate students in lecture halls, or build communities in our neighborhoods, our mission remains absolute: to protect human dignity, foster radical empathy, and ensure that the sacred worth of every individual is never compromised, never ignored, and forever defended.

The Eternal Flame of Conscience

To dwell in the spirit of "Never Again" is to accept that the defense of human dignity requires eternal, unbroken vigilance. History has demonstrated beyond doubt that cruelty thrives in the shadows of oversight, and that injustice gains ground whenever good people assume that someone else will speak up.

Let this realization anchor our daily lives and professional practices. Whether facing the pressures of modern healthcare systems, the complexities of institutional policies, or the quiet moments of interpersonal interaction, we choose to remain awake. We choose to see the human being behind every statistic, to honor the sacred worth of every life, and to keep the promise of "Never Again" alive through relentless empathy, moral courage, and unwavering love.

The Solid Battle Cry: Reclaiming Humanity from the Legacy of Human Exhibits

When the philosophy of "Never Again" is anchored directly to the dark history of human exhibits—the nineteenth and early twentieth-century spectacles where indigenous peoples, colonized individuals, disabled persons, and marginalized humans were displayed in cages, ethnographic villages, and medical sideshows for public curiosity—it transforms into an uncompromising battle cry.

In this specific historical context, the solid battle cry of "Never Again" declares:

A Human Being Is Never a Specimen: It is an absolute rejection of objectification that turns living, breathing souls into scientific curiosities, data points, or entertainment. It asserts that human worth is intrinsic, sacred, and entirely divorced from utility, novelty, or aesthetic value.

The Demanding Call to Restitution and Recognition: It demands that the historical victims of exhibitionism—such as Saartjie Baartman (the Hottentot Venus) and countless unnamed individuals whose remains and dignity were commodified—be honored with truth, profound respect, and the full restoration of their humanity.

The Modern Firewall Against Clinical and Social Exhibitionism: For modern professionals—especially nurses and frontline clinicians—this battle cry echoes at the bedside and in research laboratories. It means ensuring that vulnerable patients are never treated as mere teaching props, diagnostic puzzles, or administrative metrics for institutional prestige.

The solid battle cry of "Never Again" in relation to human exhibits is a vow that no human being will ever again be stripped of their autonomy, put on display, or reduced to an object of curiosity. It is an eternal declaration that every person walks the earth with absolute dignity, fully protected from exploitation, indifference, and the cold gaze of voyeurism.

The Unbroken Chain of Human Responsibility

As we reflect upon the long journey through historical memory, systemic vulnerability, and the sacred vocation of nursing, the mandate of "Never Again" reveals itself as an unbreakable chain linking every generation to the next. The choices we make today, whether to challenge indifference, to protect the vulnerable, or to stand firm against institutional apathy—form the foundation upon which tomorrow's world is built.

Let us carry this responsibility forward with unyielding courage and boundless compassion. In every classroom, every boardroom, every laboratory, and every quiet hospital room, we remain the guardians of the human spirit. The promise of "Never Again" is not merely words on a page; it is a living, breathing commitment to honor the absolute, inviolable worth of every human being—today, tomorrow, and for all eternity.

The Polyphonic Voice of "Never Again"

To fully comprehend the mandate of "Never Again," we must listen to how this sacred vow echoes across the distinct pillars of human society. It is not spoken in a single tone; rather, it is a polyphonic chorus rising from healthcare, education, research, and everyday life, each domain bearing a unique responsibility to protect human dignity.

The Voice of Healthcare: "Never again shall a human being be reduced to a diagnosis code, a financial asset, or an administrative burden. At the bedside, in the emergency department, and in the quietest hours of palliative care, we vow that clinical efficiency shall never eclipse sacred worth. We stand as the human firewall against apathy, ensuring that vulnerability is met with fierce, unconditional compassion.

The Voice of Education: "Never again shall classrooms or lecture halls breed silent complicity. We commit to teaching the brutal honesty of history not as distant lore, but as a mirror for the present. We empower the next generation to interrogate structural inequality, question unjust authority, and practice the moral courage that transforms passive learners into active guardians of justice."

The Voice of Research: "Never again shall the pursuit of scientific progress or academic prestige march over the bodies and autonomy of human beings. We vow that inquiry will be guided by radical ethics, informed consent, and profound respect for personhood. Curiosity must never be weaponized into objectification; discovery is meaningless if it desecrates human dignity."

The Voice of Everyday Life: "Never again shall we look away from the stranger in need, tolerate casual prejudice in the breakroom, or mistake silence for neutrality. In our homes, our neighborhoods, and our daily interactions, we recognize that massive indifference is born of small, unchecked compromises. We choose radical empathy, holding fast to the truth that every individual matters infinitely."

The Harmonic Convergence of Human Dignity

When these four distinct voices—healthcare, education, research, and everyday life—converge, they form an impenetrable shield around the sacred worth of humanity. The vow of "Never Again" ceases to be a distant historical aspiration and becomes an active, breathing reality woven into the very fabric of our daily existence.

Whether we are holding a patient's hand in the dim light of a hospital room, mentoring a student to question injustice, ensuring ethical boundaries in a scientific laboratory, or simply choosing kindness in a quiet neighborhood interaction, we are answering the call. The work of protecting humanity is never finished, but as long as we speak with one united, unwavering voice, the promise of "Never Again" remains our unbreakable legacy.

The Voice of the Humanities Around the World

"Never again shall human suffering be translated into mere data, forgotten in the archives of time, or erased by the victors of power. Through poetry, narrative, philosophy, and art, we commit to preserving the unvarnished truth of human experience—both our deepest tragedies and our highest triumphs. We are the keepers of memory, reminding the world that empathy is born when we recognize ourselves in the face of the other. We vow to interrogate injustice, give language to the silenced, and ensure that the creative spirit of humanity remains an eternal testament to freedom, resilience, and uncompromised dignity across the globe."

The Neurobiology of Apathy and the Clinical Anatomy of Dehumanization

When the mandate of "Never Again" is examined through the rigorous lenses of advanced medicine and neuropsychology, the historical descent into systemic atrocity reveals a chilling biological substrate. Dehumanization is not merely an abstract moral failure; it is a neurological and psychological hijacking of human empathy circuits.

Neuroimaging studies demonstrate that when human beings perceive others as belonging to an "out-group" or as objects of lesser utility, the medial prefrontal cortex—the region responsible for mentalizing, perspective-taking, and recognizing personhood—shows a marked reduction in activation. In clinical environments, administrative burnout, chronic moral distress, and extreme institutional pressures can trigger this exact defensive neural shutdown. Clinicians and researchers under siege begin to unconsciously utilize psychological numbing as a defense mechanism against overwhelming stress, slowly transforming sentient patients into mere diagnostic categories, data entries, or logistical obstacles.

The Psychopathology of Compliance and the Banality of Cruelty

Psychologically, the roots of historical medical abuse and institutional apathy lie in the complex interplay of authority, obedience, and cognitive dissonance. Milgram's classic paradigms and subsequent psychiatric evaluations of institutional compliance reveal how easily professional socialization can override individual moral agency. When healthcare workers, scientists, or educators are embedded within hierarchical systems that prioritize institutional utility over human welfare, dangerous psychological compartmentalization occurs.

Under these conditions, individuals disown their personal moral authorship:

Diffusion of Responsibility: The psychological burden of ethical failure is distributed across the entire institutional machinery, allowing perpetrators and passive observers alike to feel personally blameless.

Euphemistic Labeling: Human suffering is clinically sanitized through bureaucratic language—such as "resource allocation," "triage optimization," or "experimental cohorts"—which severs the emotional connection between the clinician's action and the patient's visceral reality.

Moral Injury as a Diagnostic Warning: Conversely, when healthcare professionals are forced to participate in or witness systems that violate human dignity, they experience profound moral injury—a psychological trauma characterized by deep guilt, existential despair, and the shattering of their fundamental trust in professional ethics.

The Neurological Architecture of Radical Empathy

To enact "Never Again" at a clinical and psychological level requires building an active neurological and emotional counterweight to apathy. Empathy is not a finite, exhaustible emotion; it is an intentionally cultivated cognitive and affective capacity rooted in mirror neuron activation, affective resonance, and executive cognitive regulation.

In the high-stakes crucible of healthcare, psychological resilience must be reframed. True resilience is not the ability to withstand institutional exploitation or harden oneself against patient suffering; rather, it is the fierce, daily psychological discipline of remaining soft-hearted in hard places. It is the conscious activation of empathy through reflective practice, clinical debriefing, interprofessional peer support, and structural advocacy.

By treating empathy as a vital clinical vital sign—as essential to patient survival as blood pressure or oxygen saturation, the modern medical and scientific community establishes an impenetrable psychological defense. We recognize that to protect the human body, we must relentlessly protect the human psyche, ensuring that the sacred boundary of personhood is never breached by convenience, fatigue, or fear.

The Visceral Somatics of Suffering: The Body Remembers What the Institution Forgets

When the philosophy of "Never Again" descends from abstract ethics into the raw, visceral domain of the human body, it confronts the undeniable truth that trauma, dignity, and neglect are physically inscribed into human tissue. The body is not a detached vessel or a mechanical assembly of organ systems; it is the living archive of human experience.

In clinical and psychological spaces, when a patient is reduced to a diagnosis code, a statistical outlier, or an administrative metric, the somatic consequence is profound. Chronic stress, institutional betrayal, and medical marginalization trigger sustained activation of the hypothalamic-pituitary-adrenal (HPA) axis, flooding the body with cortisol and catecholamines. Over time, this biological wear and tear—known as allostatic load—alters neurological wiring, suppresses immune function, and imprints deep somatic memories of powerlessness.

To practice "Never Again" at a physical level means recognizing that healing requires more than pharmacological intervention; it demands the restoration of bodily safety. It requires a clinician to look past clinical detachment and perceive the physiological language of distress: the shallow breath of a terrified patient, the guarded posture of someone whose autonomy has been compromised, or the silent tremor of an individual who has learned that the healthcare system is a place of vulnerability rather than sanctuary.

The Intimate Micro-Kinetics of Compassionate Touch

At the absolute frontier of human touch, the nursing spirit enacts physical counterweight to historical apathy. Physical touch in a clinical setting is never neutral; it is either an act of mechanical objectification or a radical gesture of human restoration.

Imagine the somatic reality of a bedside interaction where touch communicates absolute worth:

The Grounding Touch: When a nurse places a warm, steady hand on the shoulder of a patient experiencing acute medical panic or gently holds the arm of an elderly individual navigating profound disorientation, sensory receptors transmit immediate signals of safety to the limbic system, downregulating the neurobiological alarm bells of fear.

The Reassertion of Ownership: For individuals who carry historical or institutional trauma—where their physical forms were once treated as specimens, subjects, or burdens—gentle, respectful, and consent-driven touch restores agency over their own bodies. It declares unequivocally: This body belongs to you. Your physical form is sacred, inviolable, and worthy of profound tenderness.

The Emotional Depth of Relational Resonance

Psychologically, true empathy is not a passive observation of another's pain; it is a profound emotional resonance willingness to enter the dark, quiet chambers of a patient's existential suffering without turning away.

When a clinician allows themselves to emotionally co-regulate with a suffering human being, they bridge the artificial gulf that institutions build between "the professional" and "the patient." This emotional depth requires extraordinary courage, because it exposes the clinician to the raw grief, anger, and fear of the human condition. Yet, it is precisely this shared emotional weight that prevents the recurrence of institutional coldness.

When we honor the physical and emotional reality of "Never Again," we acknowledge that human dignity is a shared biological and psychological state. We bind our nervous systems to the cause of justice, ensuring that every touch heals, every presence validates, and every breath we draw in service to others is a living defense of the sacred human spirit.

The Voice of Humanitarian Law

To weave the ultimate boundary around human dignity, we must listen to the stern, unyielding voice of international humanitarian law, the global codification of conscience born from the ashes of history's darkest atrocities:

"Never again shall state sovereignty, military necessity, or bureaucratic convenience be invoked to justify the suspension of human worth. Through the Geneva Conventions, international criminal tribunals, and universal human rights frameworks, we declare that certain acts are inherently intolerable, eternally unlawful, and universally condemned. We bind nations and individuals alike to the absolute duty of protection—guaranteeing that even in the chaos of war, displacement, and systemic crisis, the vulnerable are shielded, the perpetrator of atrocities is held accountable, and the sacred law of humanity remains supreme across every border on earth."

The Voice of the Author

As the final words of this volume settle into silence, the author steps back from the text to speak directly to you, the reader, across the bridge of our shared humanity.

"When I set out to write these pages, the mandate of 'Never Again' was not merely an academic exercise or a historical retrospective; it was a deeply personal plea and an urgent moral summons. I wrote this because history has shown us, with terrifying clarity, that the descent into indifference never happens overnight. It begins in the quietest corners of our minds, the unexamined biases in our breakrooms, the systemic shortcuts in our institutions, and the moments when we choose comfort over courage.

As an author, my ultimate hope is that these chapters do not rest quietly on a shelf as a monument to tragedies past, but that they become a living, breathing pulse within your own conscience.

Whether you are a nurse holding a hand at a bedside, a student questioning the status quo, a researcher guarding the sacred boundaries of ethics, or a neighbor choosing empathy in a fractured world, the responsibility now rests in your hands. Never again let suffering be met with silence. Never again let a human being be reduced to statistics. Carry this vow forward into every room you enter, every choice you make, and every life you touch. The future of human dignity belongs to those who refuse to look away."

The Final Cadence: An Unbroken Legacy

The journey through history, healthcare ethics, somatic trauma, scientific responsibility, global humanities, international law, and personal conscience has led us to a singular, luminous realization: the promise of "Never Again" is not a destination we finally reach, but an eternal fire we must forever tend.

We have traced the terrifying mechanics of how atrocities are born—not from sudden, monstrous explosions, but from the slow, quiet erosion of empathy, the weaponization of efficiency, and the dangerous luxury of looking away. We have witnessed how easily human beings can be reduced to data points, diagnostic codes, or objects of curiosity, and how institutional apathy creates the fertile soil in which cruelty takes root.

Yet, we have also witnessed the indomitable power of the human spirit.

We have heard the nursing voice declaring the bedside an inviolable sanctuary of unconditional worth and radical presence.

We have felt the somatic and psychological reality of trauma, recognizing that physical touch and emotional resonance are profound acts of resistance against the machinery of indifference.

We have listened to the voices of education, research, and everyday life, reminding us that moral courage belongs to every single one of us in our daily choices.

We have absorbed the solemn decrees of humanitarian law, binding nations and individuals to the absolute duty of universal protection.

And finally, we have carried the humanities and the author's personal plea, transforming historical memory into a living compass for the future.

The work is never finished. Every sunrise brings a new opportunity to choose empathy over apathy, justice over convenience, and courage over fear.

Carry this vow forward into the hospitals, the classrooms, the laboratories, the legislative halls, and the quiet streets of your communities. Be the voice for the silenced, the shield for the vulnerable, and the unwavering guardian of human dignity.

Let the past be your teacher, let your conscience be your guide, and let the promise of "Never Again" remain your unbreakable shield—today, tomorrow, and for all generations to come.

BIBLIOGRAPHY

Agamben, Giorgio. 1998. *Homo Sacer: Sovereign Power and Bare Life*. Stanford: Stanford University Press.

———. 2005. *State of Exception*. Chicago: University of Chicago Press.

Agoncillo, Teodoro A. 1956. *The Revolt of the Masses: The Story of Bonifacio and the Katipunan*. Quezon City: University of the Philippines Press.

Allport, Gordon W. 1954. *The Nature of Prejudice*. Cambridge, MA: Addison-Wesley.

American Nurses Association. 2015. *Code of Ethics for Nurses with Interpretive Statements*. Silver Spring, MD: American Nurses Association.

Arendt, Hannah. 1951. *The Origins of Totalitarianism*. New York: Schocken Books.

———. 1963. *Eichmann in Jerusalem: A Report on the Banality of Evil*. New York: Viking Press.

Achebe, Chinua. 1958. *Things Fall Apart*. London: Heinemann.

Bandura, Albert. 1999. "Moral Disengagement in the Perpetration of Inhumanities." *Personality and Social Psychology Review* 3 (3): 193–209.

Bauman, Zygmunt. 1989. *Modernity and the Holocaust*. Cambridge: Polity Press.

Beauchamp, Tom L., and James F. Childress. 2019. *Principles of Biomedical Ethics*. 8th ed. New York: Oxford University Press.

Beecher, Henry K. 1966. "Ethics and Clinical Research." *New England Journal of Medicine* 274 (24): 1354–60.

Benedict, Ruth. 1983. *The Anthropology of St. Louis: Displaying the Primitive at the 1904 World's Fair*. Urbana: University of Illinois Press.

Bhatt, Ambrish. 2010. "Evolution of Clinical Research: A History Before and Beyond James Lind." *Perspectives in Clinical Research* 1 (1): 6–6. https://doi.org/10.4103/2229-3485.71839.

Bourgeois, Philippe. 2003. *In Search of Respect: Selling Crack in El Barrio*. Cambridge: Cambridge University Press.

Bourgois, Philippe, and Jeff Schonberg. 2009. *Righteous Dopefiend*. Berkeley: University of California Press.

Bourne, Russell. 2001. *Exhibiting Empire: Anthropology and the 1904 Louisiana Purchase Exposition*. Lincoln: University of Nebraska Press.

Butler, Judith. 2004. *Precarious Life: The Powers of Mourning and Violence*. London: Verso.

Camus, Albert. 1947. *The Plague*. New York: Alfred A. Knopf.

Canguilhem, Georges. 1991. *The Normal and the Pathological*. New York: Zone Books.

Cassel, Eric J. 1982. "The Nature of Suffering and the Goals of Medicine." *New England Journal of Medicine* 306 (11): 639–45.

Cikara, Mina, Emile G. Bruneau, and Rebecca R. Saxe. 2011. "Us and Them: Intergroup Failures of Empathy." *Current Directions in Psychological Science* 20 (3): 149–53.

Coates, Ta-Nehisi. 2015. *Between the World and Me*. New York: Spiegel & Grau.

Cole, Harry M. 2006. "Medical Ethics and Human Experimentation: Historical Reflections." *Journal of Medical Ethics* 32 (4): 210–15.

Constantino, Renato. 1975. *The Philippines: A Past Revisited.* Quezon City: Tala Publishing Services.

Coronel, Sheila S., ed. 1998. *The Rulemakers: How the Wealthy and Well-Born Influence Lawmaking*. Quezon City: Philippine Center for Investigative Journalism.

Crenshaw, Kimberlé. 1995. *Critical Race Theory: The Key Writings That Formed the Movement*. New York: The New Press.

Cruz, Fernando A. 2018. "Institutional Memory, Archival Preservation, and Historical Trauma in Philippine Repositories." *Philippine Social Sciences Review* 70 (2): 45–68.

Davis, Angela Y. 2003. *Are Prisons Obsolete?* New York: Seven Stories Press.

De la Costa, Horacio. 1961. *The Jesuits in the Philippines, 1581–1768*. Cambridge, MA: Harvard University Press.

Desjarlais, Robert. 1997. *Shelter Blues: Sanity and Selfhood Among the Homeless*. Philadelphia: University of Pennsylvania Press.

De Waal, Frans. 2009. *The Age of Empathy: Nature's Lessons for a Kinder Society*. New York: Crown.

Dunbar, Robin I. M. 2016. *Human Evolution: Our Brains and Behavior*. Oxford: Oxford University Press.

Eagleton, Terry. 2003. *Sweet Violence: The Idea of the Tragic*. Oxford: Blackwell Publishing.

Eban, Abba. 1983. *The New Diplomacy: International Affairs in the Modern Age*. New York: Random House.

Fanon, Frantz. 1952. *Black Skin, White Masks*. Paris: Éditions du Seuil.

———. 1961. *The Wretched of the Earth*. Paris: Présence Africaine.

Farmer, Paul. 2003. *Pathologies of Power: Health, Human Rights, and the New War on the Poor*. Berkeley: University of California Press.

Fassin, Didier. 2011. *Humanitarian Reason: A Moral History of the Present*. Berkeley: University of California Press.

Fletcher, Joseph. 1967. "Human Experimentation: Ethics in the Consent Situation." *Law and Contemporary Problems* 32 (4): 620–40. https://doi.org/10.2307/1190856.

Fontesse, Sarah, Stéphanie Demoulin, Fabrice Stinglhamber, Paul De Timary, and Pierre Maurage. 2021. "Metadehumanization and Self-Dehumanization Are Linked to Reduced Drinking Refusal

Self-Efficacy and Increased Anxiety and Depression Symptoms in Patients with Severe Alcohol Use Disorder." *Psychologica Belgica* 61: 238–52. https://doi.org/10.5334/pb.1058.

Foucault, Michel. 1973. *The Birth of the Clinic: An Archaeology of Medical Perception*. London: Tavistock Publications.

Frank, Arthur W. 1995. *The Wounded Storyteller: Body, Illness, and Ethics*. Chicago: University of Chicago Press.

Frankl, Viktor E. 1946. *Man's Search for Meaning*. Boston: Beacon Press.

Freire, Paulo. 1970. *Pedagogy of the Oppressed*. New York: Herder and Herder.

Fromm, Erich. 1973. *The Anatomy of Human Destructiveness*. New York: Holt, Rinehart and Winston.

Fulton, Tanja, Elizabeth C. Lathan, Megan C. Karkare, Andrea Guelfo, Laleh Eghbalzad, Vibha Ahluwalia, Tanja D. Ely, et al. 2024. "Civilian Moral Injury and Amygdala Functional Connectivity During Attention to Threat." *Biological Psychiatry: Cognitive Neuroscience and Neuroimaging* 9: 112–20. https://doi.org/10.1016/j.bpsc.2023.07.006.

Giroux, Henry A. 2014. *Neoliberalism's War on Higher Education*. Chicago: Haymarket Books.

Goffman, Erving. 1961. *Asylums: Essays on the Social Situation of Mental Patients and Other Inmates*. Anchor Books.

Goleman, Daniel. 2006. *Social Intelligence: The New Science of Human Relationships*. New York: Bantam Books.

Gramsci, Antonio. 1971. *Selections from the Prison Notebooks*. New York: International Publishers.

Grosfoguel, Ramón. 2007. "The Epistemic Decolonial Turn: Beyond Political-Economy Paradigms." *Cultural Studies* 21 (2–3): 211–23. https://doi.org/10.1080/09502380601162514.

Hacking, Ian. 1986. *The Taming of Chance*. Cambridge: Cambridge University Press.

Hasso, Suhair. 2012. "Dehumanization and Clinical Ethics: A Retrospective Review." *Nursing Ethics* 19 (2): 245–59. https://doi.org/10.1177/0969733011423403.

Haslam, Nick. 2006. "Dehumanization: An Integrative Review." *Personality and Social Psychology Review* 10 (3): 252–64. https://doi.org/10.1207/s15327957pspr1003_4.

Helman, Cecil G. 2007. *Culture, Health and Illness*. 5th ed. London: Hodder Arnold.

Holmes, Seth M. 2013. *Fresh Fruit, Broken Bodies: Migrant Farmworkers in the United States*. Berkeley: University of California Press.

Hoogendoorn, Caitlin J., and Nilda D. Rodríguez. 2023. "Rethinking Dehumanization, Empathy, and Burnout in Healthcare Contexts." *Current Opinion in Behavioral Sciences* 52: 101285. https://doi.org/10.1016/j.cobeha.2023.101285.

hooks, bell. 2000. *All About Love: New Visions*. New York: William Morrow.

Humphrey, John P. 1949. "The Universal Declaration of Human Rights." *International Journal* 4 (4): 351–61. https://doi.org/10.3138/IJ.4.4.351.

Ignatieff, Michael. 2001. *Human Rights as Politics and Idolatry*. Princeton, NJ: Princeton University Press.

Iliffe, John. 1987. *The African Poor: A History*. Cambridge: Cambridge University Press.

Ileto, Reynaldo C. 1979. *Pasyon and Revolution: Popular Movements in the Philippines, 1840–1910*. Quezon City: Ateneo de Manila University Press.

International Council of Nurses. 2021. *The ICN Code of Ethics for Nurses*. Geneva: International Council of Nurses.

Ivy, Andrew C. 1948. "The History and Ethics of the Use of Human Subjects in Medical Experiments." *Science* 108 (2792): 1–5. https://doi.org/10.1126/science.108.2792.1.

Jonas, Hans. 1970. "Philosophical Reflections on Experimenting with Human Subjects." *Daedalus* 99 (2): 219–47.

———. 1984. *The Imperative of Responsibility: In Search of an Ethics for the Technological Age*. Chicago: University of Chicago Press.

Kaptchuk, Ted J. 2011. "Placebo Studies and the Meaning Response: Neurobiological Implications." *Science Translational Medicine* 3 (100): 100cm43. https://doi.org/10.1126/scitranslmed.3000297.

Kelman, Herbert C. 1973. "Violence Without Moral Restraint: Reflections on the Dehumanization of Victims and Victimizers." *Journal of Social Issues* 29 (4): 25–61. https://doi.org/10.1111/j.1540-4560.1973.tb00103.x.

Kendi, Ibram X. 2019. *How to Be an Antiracist*. New York: One World.

Kierkegaard, Søren. 1844. *The Concept of Anxiety*. Princeton, NJ: Princeton University Press.

Kleinman, Arthur. 1988. *The Illness Narratives: Suffering, Healing, And The Human Condition*. New York: Basic Books.

Kramer, Paul A. 2006. *The Blood of Government: Race, Empire, the United States, and the Philippines*. Chapel Hill: University of North Carolina Press.

Kristeva, Julia. 1982. *Powers of Horror: An Essay on Abjection*. New York: Columbia University Press.

Latour, Bruno. 1987. *Science in Action: How to Follow Scientists and Engineers Through Society*. Cambridge, MA: Harvard University Press.

Lears, T. J. Jackson. 1994. *No Place of Grace: Antimodernism and the Transformation of American Culture, 1880–1920*. Chicago: University of Chicago Press.

Levi, Primo. 1986. *If This Is a Man / The Truce*. London: Penguin Books.

Levinas, Emmanuel. 1969. *Totality and Infinity: An Essay on Exteriority*. Pittsburgh: Duquesne University Press.

Lifton, Robert Jay. 1986. *The Nazi Doctors: Medical Killing and the Psychology of Genocide*. New York: Basic Books.

Lorde, Audre. 1984. *Sister Outsider: Essays and Speeches*. Trumansburg, NY: Crossing Press.

Mamdani, Mahmood. 1996. *Citizen and Subject: Contemporary Africa and the Legacy of Late Colonialism*. Princeton, NJ: Princeton University Press.

May, Larry. 1987. *The Morality of Groups: Collective Responsibility, Group-Based Harm, and Corporate Morality*. Notre Dame, IN: University of Notre Dame Press.

Mbembe, Achille. 2001. *On the Postcolony*. Berkeley: University of California Press.

———. 2019. *Necropolitics*. Durham, NC: Duke University Press.

McCoy, Alfred W., ed. 1994. *An Anarchy of Families: State and Family in the Philippines*. Quezon City: Ateneo de Manila University Press.

McCrudden, Christopher. 2022. "Human Dignity." In *Elgar Encyclopedia of Human Rights*, 430–39. Cheltenham: Edward Elgar Publishing. https://doi.org/10.4337/9781789903621.human.dignity.

Mead, George Herbert. 1934. *Mind, Self and Society*. Chicago: University of Chicago Press.

Memmi, Albert. 1965. *The Colonizer and the Colonized*. New York: Orion Press.

Mendez, Mario F. 2022. "A Functional and Neuroanatomical Model of Dehumanization." *Cognitive and Behavioral Neurology* 36 (1): 42–47. https://doi.org/10.1097/wnn.0000000000000316.

Merleau-Ponty, Maurice. 1945. *Phenomenology of Perception*. London: Routledge.

Milgram, Stanley. 1974. *Obedience to Authority: An Experimental View*. New York: Harper & Row.

Minow, Martha. 1998. *Between Vengeance and Forgiveness: Facing History After Genocide and Mass Violence*. Boston: Beacon Press.

Mitscherlich, Alexander, and Fred Mielke. 1949. *Doctors of Infamy: The Story of the Nazi Medical Crimes*. New York: Henry Schuman.

Montgomery, Kathryn. 2006. *How Doctors Think: Clinical Judgment and the Practice of Medicine*. Oxford: Oxford University Press.

Mumford, Lewis. 1967. *The Myth of the Machine: Technics and Human Development*. New York: Harcourt, Brace & World.

National Historical Commission of the Philippines. 2012. *The Documentation and Archival Preservation of Wartime Atrocities and Medical Experiments in Manila, 1941–1945*. Manila: NHCP Archives.

Nietzsche, Friedrich. 1887. *On the Genealogy of Morality*. Oxford: Oxford University Press.

Nussbaum, Martha C. 2001. *Upheavals of Thought: The Intelligence of Emotions*. Cambridge: Cambridge University Press.

———. 2010. *Not for Profit: Why Democracy Needs the Humanities*. Princeton, NJ: Princeton University Press.

———. 2011. *Creating Capabilities: The Human Development Approach*. Cambridge, MA: Harvard University Press.

Orwell, George. 1949. *Nineteen Eighty-Four*. London: Secker & Warburg.

Packard, Randall M. 1989. *White Plague, Black Labor: Tuberculosis and the Political Economy of Health and Disease in South Africa*. Berkeley: University of California Press.

Pearsall, Tamara. 2001. *The Subject of Human Exhibition: Spectacle and Subalternity in the Nineteenth Century*. Durham, NC: Duke University Press.

Perkins, Brian I. 2020. "Health Care Today: Whom Do We Really Care About?" *Linacre Quarterly* 88 (1): 32–36. https://doi.org/10.1177/0024363920951660.

Pfohl, Stephen. 2009. *Critical Sociology: Towards an End of the Normal*. Dix Hills, NY: General Hall.

Polanyi, Karl. 1944. *The Great Transformation: The Political and Economic Origins of Our Time*. New York: Farrar & Rinehart.

Popper, Steven E., and Kent McCloskey. 1995. "Ethics in Human Experimentation: Historical Perspectives." *Military Medicine* 160 (1): 7–11. https://doi.org/10.1093/milmed/160.1.7.

Purtilo, Ruth B., and Regina F. Doherty. 2011. *Ethical Dimensions in the Health Professions*. 5th ed. St. Louis: Saunders.

Quibuyen, Floro C. 1999. *A Nation Aborted: Rizal, American Hegemony, and Philippine Nationalism*. Quezon City: Ateneo de Manila University Press.

Rafael, Vicente L. 1988. *Contracting Colonialism: Translation and Christian Conversion in Tagalog Society Under Early Spanish Rule*. Ithaca, NY: Cornell University Press.

Rancière, Jacques. 2004. *The Politics of Aesthetics*. London: Continuum.

Rawls, John. 1971. *A Theory of Justice*. Cambridge, MA: Harvard University Press.

Reyes, Pia Angela. 2020. "Bioethics and Historical Vulnerabilities: Medical Research Ethics in Post-Colonial Philippine Healthcare Settings." *Asian Bioethics Review* 12 (3): 289–304. https://doi.org/10.1007/s41649-020-00134-y.

Rizzolatti, Giacomo, and Corrado Craighero. 2004. "The Mirror-Neuron System." *Annual Review of Neuroscience* 27: 169–92. https://doi.org/10.1146/annurev.neuro.27.070203.144230.

Rodney, Walter. 1972. *How Europe Underdeveloped Africa*. London: Bogle-L'Ouverture Publications.

Rose, Nikolas. 2007. *The Politics of Life Itself: Biomedicine, Power, and Subjectivity in the Twenty-First Century*. Princeton, NJ: Princeton University Press.

Roupa, Anastasia, Areti Patelarou, Evridiki C. Fradelos, Konstantina Fousiani, Marina Miliaraki, Konstantinos Giakoumidakis, and Evangelos Patelarou. 2024. "Validation of Two Instruments for the Measurement of Dehumanization and Self-Dehumanization in Healthcare Settings." *Nursing Reports* 14 (3): 2246–65. https://doi.org/10.3390/nursrep14030167.

Roy, Arundhati. 2001. *The Cost of Living*. New York: Modern Library.

Rydell, Robert W. 1984. *All the World's a Fair: Visions of Empire at American International Expositions, 1876–1916*. Chicago: University of Chicago Press.

Said, Edward W. 1978. *Orientalism*. New York: Pantheon Books.

Sartre, Jean-Paul. 1943. *Being and Nothingness*. New York: Philosophical Library.

Saul, John S. 2006. *Development Without Freedom: The Politics of Economic Liberation in South Africa*. London: Zed Books.

Scarry, Elaine. 1985. *The Body in Pain: The Making and Unmaking of the World*. New York: Oxford University Press.

Scheper-Hughes, Nancy. 1992. *Death Without Weeping: The Violence of Everyday Life in Brazil*. Berkeley: University of California Press.

Schumacher, John N. 1981. *Revolutionary Clergy: The Filipino Clergy and the Nationalist Movement, 1850–1903*. Quezon City: Ateneo de Manila University Press.

Sen, Amartya. 1999. *Development as Freedom*. Oxford: Oxford University Press.

Shelton, Dinah L. 2007. "An Introduction to the History of International Human Rights Law." *SSRN Electronic Journal*. https://doi.org/10.2139/ssrn.1010489.

Shklar, Judith N. 1984. *Ordinary Vices*. Cambridge, MA: Harvard University Press.

Simon, Jennifer C., and Julie N. Gutsell. 2021. "Recognizing Humanity: Dehumanization Predicts Neural Mirroring and Empathic Accuracy in Face-to-Face Interactions." *Social Cognitive and Affective Neuroscience* 16 (5): 463–73. https://doi.org/10.1093/scan/nsab014.

Sloterdijk, Peter. 1987. *Critique of Cynical Reason*. Minneapolis: University of Minnesota Press.

Sontag, Susan. 2003. *Regarding the Pain of Others*. New York: Farrar, Straus and Giroux.

Spiegel, Marjorie. 1996. *The Dreaded Comparison: Human and Animal Slavery*. New York: Mirror Books.

Spiegelman, Art. 1986. *Maus: A Survivor's Tale*. New York: Pantheon Books.

Stanley, Peter W. 1974. *A Nation in the Making: The Philippines and the United States, 1899–1921*. Cambridge, MA: Harvard University Press.

Stengers, Isabelle. 2010. *Cosmopolitics I*. Minneapolis: University of Minnesota Press.

Stoler, Ann Laura. 2002. *Carnal Knowledge and Imperial Power: Race and the Intimate in Colonial Rule*. Berkeley: University of California Press.

Tajfel, Henri, and John C. Turner. 1979. "An Integrative Theory of Intergroup Conflict." In *The Social Psychology of Intergroup Relations*, edited by William G. Austin and Stephen Worchel, 33–47. Monterey, CA: Brooks/Cole.

Tan, Michael L. 2008. *Revisiting Healing Arts: The Politics of Health and Medicine in the Philippines*. Quezon City: University of the Philippines Press.

Taylor, Charles. 1989. *Sources of the Self: The Making of the Modern Identity*. Cambridge, MA: Harvard University Press.

Tillich, Paul. 1952. *The Courage to Be*. New Haven, CT: Yale University Press.

Todorov, Tzvetan. 1996. *Facing the Extreme: Moral Life in the Concentration Camps*. New York: Metropolitan Books.

United Nations. 1948. *Universal Declaration of Human Rights*. New York: United Nations General Assembly.

United Nations Educational, Scientific and Cultural Organization. 1997. *Universal Declaration on the Human Genome and Human Rights*. Paris: UNESCO.

Van der Kolk, Bessel A. 2014. *The Body Keeps the Score: Brain, Mind, and Body in the Healing of Trauma*. New York: Viking.

Varzi, Achille C. 2003. "The Nature of Spatial and Temporal Boundaries." *Stanford Encyclopedia of Philosophy*.

Vaughan, Megan. 1991. *Curing Their Ills: Colonial Power and African Illness*. Cambridge: Polity Press.

Vergès, Françoise. 1998. *Monsters and Revolutionaries: Colonial Family Romance and Métissage*. Durham, NC: Duke University Press.

Walzer, Michael. 1977. *Just and Unjust Wars: A Moral Argument with Historical Illustrations*. New York: Basic Books.

Wacquant, Loïc. 2009. *Punishing the Poor: The Neoliberal Government of Social Insecurity*. Durham, NC: Duke University Press.

Weber, Max. 1946. *From Max Weber: Essays in Sociology*. Translated and edited by H. H. Gerth and C. Wright Mills. New York: Oxford University Press.

Weil, Simone. 1952. *The Need for Roots: Prelude to a Declaration of Duties Towards Mankind*. London: Routledge.

White, Richard W. 1999. *The Moral Imagination: Case Studies in Ethics and Leadership*. San Francisco: Jossey-Bass.

Wiesel, Elie. 1960. *Night*. New York: Hill and Wang.

Williams, Bernard. 1985. *Ethics and the Limits of Philosophy*. Cambridge, MA: Harvard University Press.

Wolff, Robert Paul. 1970. *In Defense of Anarchism*. New York: University of California Press.

World Medical Association. 2013. "WMA Declaration of Helsinki: Ethical Principles for Medical Research Involving Human Subjects." *JAMA* 310 (20): 2191–94. https://doi.org/10.1001/jama.2013.281053.

Young, Iris Marion. 1990. *Justice and the Politics of Difference*. Princeton, NJ: Princeton University Press.

Zimbardo, Philip. 2007. *The Lucifer Effect: Understanding How Good People Turn Evil*. New York: Random House.

ABOUT THE AUTHOR

Richard Logro, Ph.D., RN is a versatile writer whose catalog spans vital healthcare non-fiction, an impactful nursing trilogy, historical inquiry, and imaginative children's literature. Driven by a passion for storytelling and compassionate care, his work has earned international acclaim, notably with the opening volume of his signature nursing trilogy, The Story of Filipino Nurses Around the Globe, being named a 2026 International Ebobea Book Awards Finalist. The trilogy continues with The Healer's Genesis and The Stoic Nurse, complemented by his whimsical children's adventure The Tale of the Little Surgeon and the Whispering Woods. Balancing a day-to-day career as a public health and community school nurse with a prolific publishing schedule, Richard continues to champion education and storytelling from his home in Maryland.

www.ingramcontent.com/pod-product-compliance
Lightning Source LLC
LaVergne TN
LVHW050754061126
851857LV00012B/553
* 9 7 9 8 1 8 2 7 2 0 5 1 9 *